# Black's
# CONCISE ATLAS OF
# HUMAN ANATOMY

D0412875

**KENT LIBRARIES AND ARCHIVES**

C 153663321

Askews

First edition 2005
A&C Black Publishers Ltd
37 Soho Square
London W1D 3QZ
www.acblack.com

ISBN 0–7136–7234–X

Published by arrangement with Anatographica, LLC

Text copyright © 2005 by Anatographica, LLC
Design copyright © by Anatographica, LLC

All digital Anatomy images copyright © 1999, 2001, 2003, 2004, 2005 by Visible Productions, LLC

LifeART images on pages 40, 41, and 95 copyright © 1999, 2000 Lippincott Williams & Wilkins. All rights reserved

Visible Human Project™ is a trademark of the National Library of Medicine

A CIP catalogue record for this book is available from the British Library

All rights reserved. No part of this publication may be reproduced in any form or by any means – graphic, electronic or mechanical, including photocopying, recording, taping, or information storage and retrieval systems – without the prior permission in writing of the publishers.

General Editor:          Thomas O. McCracken, MS
                              VP, Visible Productions, LLC, Fort Collins, Colorado

Senior writer:           Jim Glenn

Editor:                   Ali Moore
Art director:            Peter Laws
Designer:               Phoebe Wong
Anatomy consultant:    Dr John Lucocq MB BCh BSc PhD

Designed, edited, and typeset by Anatographica, LLC

Printed and bound in Singapore

07 D2 5 4 3 2

Black's
# CONCISE ATLAS OF
# HUMAN ANATOMY

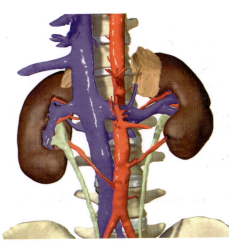

General editor: **Thomas O. McCracken**
Senior writer: **Jim Glenn**

A & C  BLACK  •  LONDON

# INTRODUCTION

With computer-aided graphics and associated modern technologies, anatomical illustration has acquired prodigious new potential. For the first time, the full body can be given a digital existence, as it were, inside the considerable and flexible processing space of a computer. This has been achieved by preparing successive thin slices of the complete body, recording them digitally, and reassembling the "stack" point-by-point with imaging software. Working from the same "dataset", accurate views can be called up to nearly any specification: a certain muscle, blood vessels in a given region, all tissues visible in a particular cross-sectional plane, an isolated organ—perhaps seen and rotated in a three-dimensional view—and so forth, filling the whole scope of imagination.

All of this has been made possible using a master dataset compiled by the Visible Human Project™ (an undertaking of the National Library of Medicine) and presented here, in the *Concise Atlas of Human Anatomy*, with the aid of graphical software developed by Visible Productions. The result is a fully accurate, fully realistic virtual anatomy, the state of the art in present-day anatomical illustration.

## Historical background

The origins of anatomical study are lost in time. Medical and anatomical knowledge advanced in uncertain ways in various societies, though it is clear that most acquired a good understanding of the body's parts and structure. In Egypt, for example, ancient practices in preparing the dead for mummification evolved a close knowledge of the body's interior. Early physicians in China also studied the body and its parts in detail.

Systematic observations are first recorded, in the West, in the 4th century BC. Aristotle (384–322 BC) apparently dissected scores of species and had reports of many more. The sciences flourished, at that time, in the Egyptian city of Alexandria; medicine and associated subjects, such as physiology and anatomy, developed in prescientific ways, sometimes in an empirical spirit, often as philosophy and lore. A Greek physician of the Roman era, Galen (AD 131–201), left the chief surviving texts. He had long experience, as a surgeon to gladiators, with practical medicine and in his later years, attending emperors, the leisure to study and accumulate the Alexandrian sources. His works, among them *The Usefulness of Parts* and *On Anatomical Procedures*, represent a pinnacle of sorts, for they remained an unchallenged authority for about 13 centuries. The great universities of Renaissance Europe taught anatomy from Galen and from Aristotle, with much hair-splitting disputation over seeming contradictions between the two masters. Dissections had become academic rituals, demonstrations performed by underlings while a professor recited from the predominant texts.

A typical illustration from the 16th-century physician Andreas Vesalius's *De Humani Corporis Fabrica*, in which the dissected corpse is displayed in a pose that suggests it is still a living, breathing human being.

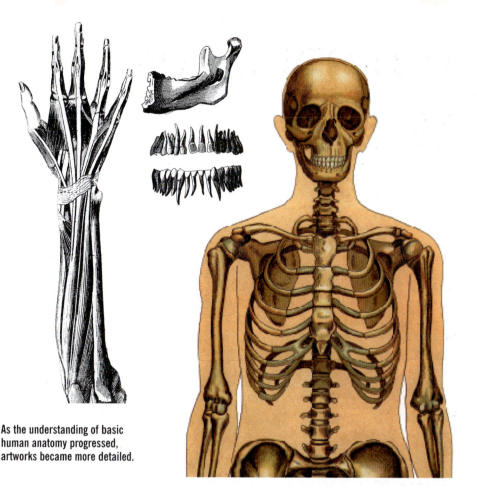

As the understanding of basic human anatomy progressed, artworks became more detailed.

A traditional anatomical depiction of the human skeleton. Such illustrations were often in themselves works of art.

With the stirrings in 16th-century Europe of a novel, scientific way of thinking, disciplines were being rebuilt. Results of this new, observational method—disseminated through a maturing printing industry—at first supplemented and then supplanted the venerated authorities in astronomy, physics, and biology. Anatomy was put on a modern footing with the publication, in 1543, of *De Humani Corporis Fabrica* ("On the Structure of the Human Body") by Andreas Vesalius (1514–1564). His detailed dissections corrected many errors transmitted in the Galenic tradition.

Other investigators were soon making important basic discoveries in physiology, among them Santorio Santorio (1561–1636; first experiments on metabolism), William Harvey (1578–1657; experimental proofs of the circulation of blood), and Giovanni Borelli (1608–1679; observations on muscle action). And as the new knowledge accumulated, at an accelerating pace through subsequent centuries, accurate illustration became an essential tool for training and instruction. Woodcuts, limited to small editions, were soon replaced by engravings and lithographic illustrations; affordable colour reproductions were introduced in the 1830s. The first edition of that most familiar reference work, Henry Gray's *Anatomy Descriptive and Surgical*, appeared in 1858.

# THE VISIBLE HUMAN PROJECT ™

Specialists in anatomy, illustrators and scientists, recognized an opportunity using digital methods to create a new, virtual anatomy. Detailed graphic information, like that contained in a photograph, can be digitized, stored, and processed in a computer. A sequence of photographs showing successive slices of some anatomical feature or region is sufficient, with the right software, to generate three-dimensional views from any chosen perspective.

A significant first effort, called the Vesalius Project, began in 1986 at Colorado State University by anatomists Thomas Spurgeon, Stephen Roper, and Thomas McCracken. In three years, the group progressed from modelling a human knee in three dimensions to a full dog's head. Images were produced by photographing individual two-dimensional views created with computerized tomography (CT) or magnetic resonance imaging (MRI). The results were somewhat low in resolution but demonstrated to striking effect the feasibility.

In 1988, at a conference of experts at the National Library of Medicine (NLM), in Bethesda, Maryland, it was decided to initiate and fund a larger endeavour, to produce a complete anatomical dataset of the body. The Visible Human Project™, as it was named, would include both a Visible Man and a Visible Woman. Charged with getting the project underway were David Whitlock and Victor Spitzer of the University of Colorado School of Medicine. Not until 1993 did they obtain their subjects, an anonymous 59-year-old woman who died of a heart blockage and a 39-year-old man, Joseph Paul Jernigan, a convict executed by lethal injection who had donated his body to science.

The Visible Man was prepared by first immobilizing the cadaver in a foaming agent, so that images could be made using various modern techniques, including X-ray, CAT, MRI, PET, and ultrasound. It was then frozen to -94°C, quartered, and embedded in a gelatin-ice mix. A precision cryomacrotome was used to cut horizontal sections 0.04 in (1 mm) thick, which were sprayed with alcohol and digitally photographed. The completed work, 1,878 colour photographs, is a (huge) dataset freely available over the internet. Converting the Visible Man into versatile 3D anatomy was yet another task, but a challenge open to anyone with the necessary theoretical and technical abilities.

## The Virtual Anatomy Project

Fortunately, another expert team had been preparing for this task since 1992. Its members had been brought together by Robert Butler, of Butler Communications, and included professors Spurgeon and McCracken—both of the ground-breaking Vesalius Project—as well as Richard Miranda (mathematics), David Alciatore (artificial intelligence and computer simulation), and Dan Steward and Chris Fredde (computer programming). The Virtual Anatomy Project began with the

The Visible Human Project™ makes it possible to produce layered images like the one above, in which the left medial wall of the nasal cavity and the left frontal sinus can clearly be seen.

welcome knowledge that a comprehensive dataset, from the Visible Human Project™, would soon be available, but a trial was performed meanwhile on 0.08-in (0.5-mm) sections of a human thorax.

The full treatment—turning sectional photos into three-dimensional virtual objects—requires that all the parts of interest be outlined, so that computer algorithms can link shapes, moving from level to level, and build the contours of three-dimensional surfaces. The linkages, point-by-point triangulations, soon grow to an unwieldy data mass and are thinned out, "decimated", by removing redundant and unnecessary points. Other algorithms are employed to add shading and texture, which produce, finally, an accurate, almost palpable image. Because all "objects" within any chosen field of view are stored as separate files, any view can be tailored—coloured or shaded, stripped of specific tissues, made transparent, rotated—at will.

Visible Productions, the organizational entity emerging from the Virtual Anatomy Project, continues to work at enlarging the capabilities of computer-aided anatomy. A logical next step involves bringing images to life, that is, endowing the body and its parts with accurate, natural motions: lungs breathing, muscles contracting, joints flexing. Using images of high precision, virtual—but highly realistic—surgery will be possible, to train students in procedures or perhaps to illustrate for patients a contemplated operation.

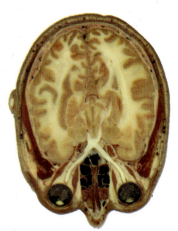

**In this horizontal (transverse) section of the head of the Visible Human, the eyes and optic nerves can clearly be seen, as can the nose and part of the ear.**

## Systemic and regional approaches

Two general approaches to anatomical illustration naturally arise. The body may be presented as it is—in depictions as close as possible artistically or photographically to what a dissector or surgeon would see as layers of tissue are removed. This is the regional approach. But it is also useful, especially for students of physiology, to represent organs more schematically, to clarify aspects of their action or operation. Organs are frequently displayed as parts of whole functional groupings, such as the digestive system, and visualized without regard to nearby, but functionally unrelated, tissues. This is the systemic approach.

Regional representation is generally the more accurate in earlier works, not least because so many of the body's systems were not yet understood or in some cases not yet even identified. Diagrammatic conceptions of, for example, the working of the heart appear as early as finely drawn regional views, but they happen to construe heart function wrongly. (The Galenic heart's left chamber, forcibly expanding, was thought to draw blood from the liver; the right side was vaguely associated with mixing air and blood.)

Both traditions, systemic and regional, remain highly useful. *Gray's Anatomy* and others in the systemic tradition are indispensable as explanatory tools. Although modern techniques can faithfully image body tissues right down to the molecular level, they seldom convey a functional sense so powerfully or clearly as does an artist's reduction of the same material. Cells, after all, are organized in ways that are not usually obvious from studying one flat, properly stained photomicrograph, or even from scrutiny of several. A crisply delineated drawing of, say, typical liver tissue reveals at one glance a complex, labyrinthine architecture—with three-dimensional features that are abstracted only from much detailed study of individual slides. On the other hand, schematic diagrams of the peripheral nervous system, no matter how clear, cannot help prepare a surgical student to find or recognize a nerve. Both approaches are helpful and, indeed, they often overlap.

# HOW TO USE THIS BOOK

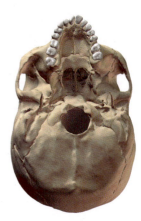

The Concise Atlas of Human Anatomy has two main sections: the first is a treatment of the body and its organs by functional system (e.g., digestion, circulation), the second an anatomical survey by physical region (e.g., arm, thorax). In systems, the longer of the two sections, organs that cooperate in carrying out a certain vital activity are described not merely by their anatomical locations—which may be dispersed around the body—but in terms of their function within a specific system. This overlaps, at a general level, with physiology, the study of how the body works. The regional section is more purely anatomical, showing parts of the body as they are situated in relation to one another.

## Terminology

Because it is a study with a rich and venerable tradition, anatomy has accumulated a large specialist vocabulary of its own. It retains a great deal of Latin and Greek in the naming of parts and systems. This provides standardization, of course, so that physicians can be quite certain about what is being described. Some of the basic terminology and underlying concepts will be outlined here; a comprehensive glossary at the end of this book is a ready reference for others, especially for those not defined elsewhere in the text. (Glossary terms are picked out in bold in the text.)

A basic need in presenting anatomical illustrations is a universal means of describing a point of view: was an artist's drawing or a CAT scan performed looking to the front? the side? from overhead? In specifying this kind of orientation, anatomists consider the body to be transected by three mutually perpendicular planes—like the x, y, and z axes of conventional algebra and three-dimensional geometry.

If the body is imagined in an upright, standing posture, a vertical plane passing through it from one side to another is termed frontal (or coronal). Vertical planes cutting across the body from front to back are medial (or sagittal). Horizontal (or transverse) planes slice at right angles to the other two. The terms "coronal" and "sagittal" refer to sutures of the skull that happen to meet at right angles and which run side-to-side (frontal bone to parietal bones) and front to back (between the parietal bones).

The planes of the body are fixed and unambiguous; they do not change if the body is flexed or positioned in some other way. It is also necessary, however, to use descriptions that can express location in a relative way: above, below, in front of, etc.

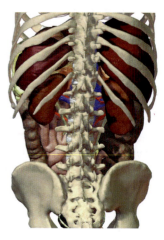

Medical terminology is very precise in its usage: the image above shows an *inferior* view of the human skull ("from below"), while the second image depicts a *posterior* ("from behind") view of the abdomen.

The most common comparative terms are:

**Anterior, posterior:** In front of (when discussing any particular view) is anterior; behind is posterior. Thus, the heart is anterior to the spine, but posterior to the sternum. Ventral (from "belly") and dorsal (from "back") mean much the same, though they refer to front and back surfaces, respectively, and are most often applied relative to the trunk or to a part that is generally thought of as having a front and back side, like the hand. Indeed, the hand is a special case, the surfaces of which are often described as palmar and dorsal; and similarly with the foot, which has plantar (of the sole) and dorsal surfaces.

**Superior, inferior:** Above is superior; below is inferior. Again, using the heart as an example, it is situated superior to the diaphragm and inferior to the aortic arch. Though not so often used, cranial (towards the head) and caudal (towards the tail) make the same distinction.

**Medial, lateral:** Towards the midline—when speaking of the body or one of its parts—is medial; away from it, to the side, is lateral. Most commonly, the body itself is the frame of reference. For example, the leg's medial surface is its inner side, towards the body's midline. In the case of the forearm, which has a naturally twisted orientation, anatomical description imagines the palm turned outward, making a medial surface along the ulna; or the distinction is often simplified, when discussing arm surfaces, in terms of its two bones, as ulnar (medial) and radial (lateral).

**Superficial, deep:** Closer to a body surface is superficial; inward, in relation to another part, is deep. Muscles, for example, often overlie one another, so the internal oblique (a middle layer of muscle in the abdominal wall) is said to be deep to the external oblique (outermost layer), but superficial to the transversus abdominis, the innermost of the three.

**Proximal, distal:** Literally, proximal means close; distal means far. For anatomical purposes, these terms are usually applied to parts that have a generally understood beginning or root, or where some part is taken to be central in a description—as for example when distinguishing arteries as proximal to (closer to) or distal to (farther from) the heart. In the case of a limb, the point of attachment to the trunk is the proximal end: the humerus articulates proximally with the scapula, distally with the ulna and radius. Proximal ends of the ulna and radius, thus, articulate with the humerus; their distal ends form a joint with the tarsals—and so on down the entire limb to the distal phalanges (last finger bones).

Median (sagittal) plane     Coronal plane

Horizontal (transverse) plane

**Specific terms are also used for the ways in which the upright human body can be dissected. The lines of division are called planes of "section".**

# CONTENTS

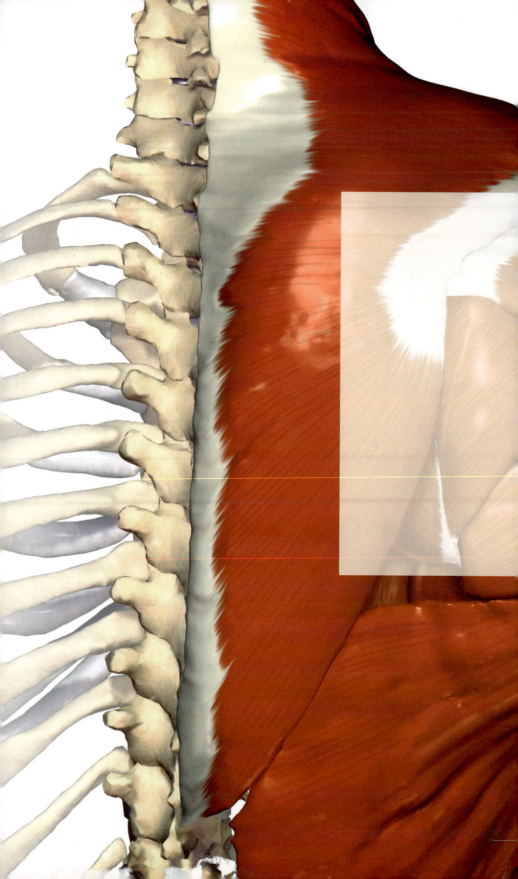

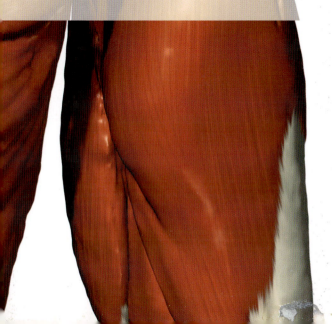

# SYSTEMIC ANATOMY

A systemic approach to anatomy looks at the human body schematically, describing how organs work as part of a whole functional grouping or system.

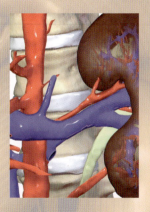

# THE INTEGUMENTARY SYSTEM

THE BODY'S OUTER COVERING, THE SKIN, is a durable, self-repairing barrier, a living 'overcoat. It also functions in regulating body temperature at around 37°C (98.6°F), whatever the ambient temperature, and provides sensory input to enable us to detect touch, pressure, pain, heat, and cold. Along with its derivatives, the hair and nails, the skin forms the body's integumentary system.

The skin has two layers, or **strata**: the epidermis, at the surface, and the dermis, just beneath it. The epidermis is constantly replacing itself; newly divided cells formed in its lowest tier, the stratum basale, are pushed gradually up to the surface, the stratum corneum, where they die and fall away.

Along the way they are transformed, filling up with **keratin** (a tough, waterproof protein) and becoming flatter so that, as they surface, reaching the stratum corneum, they make up a nonliving but protective micro-mosaic of cells.

Melanin, a brown pigment, is also produced in the lower epidermal strata; it absorbs and thus protects against the harmful ultraviolet (UV) wavelengths of sunlight.

A thicker epidermis, with five strata instead of four, is found in skin that is exposed to heavier wear, such as in the palms, fingertips, or soles of the feet. Thick skin may reach up to $\frac{3}{16}$ in (4mm) in cross-section and is always hairless. Thin skin, with a shallower epidermal region and altogether lacking the stratum lucidum, covers the rest of the body. It is hairy—with the exception of the lips and parts of the genitals.

The dermis, thicker than the epidermal layer, is stronger and more elastic—it is textured throughout with collagen and **elastin** fibres. Within the dermis are blood vessels, sensory nerve endings, sweat glands, hair follicles, and sebaceous glands. (**Sebum** is an oily substance that softens skin and aids in waterproofing.)

The hair and nails are largely formed from keratin, like the stratum corneum, and also made of dead epidermal cells, but through a different formative process that takes place in the follicles and in the nail beds. Coarse hairs, such as those on the head, are protective. Vellus, the finer, sometimes downy hair on most of the body, acts as a tactile sensor.

## Key

1. Shaft of hair
2. Stratum corneum (horny layer)
3. Stratum basale (basal layer)
4. Epidermis
5. Dermis
6. Hair follicle
7. Sebaceous gland
8. Hair bulb
9. Sweat gland
10. Duct from sweat gland
11. Stratum corneum (horny layer)
12. Stratum lucidum (clear layer)
13. Stratum granulosum (granular layer)
14. Stratum spinosum (spiny layer)
15. Dead cells flaking off from the epidermis
16. Collagen fibres

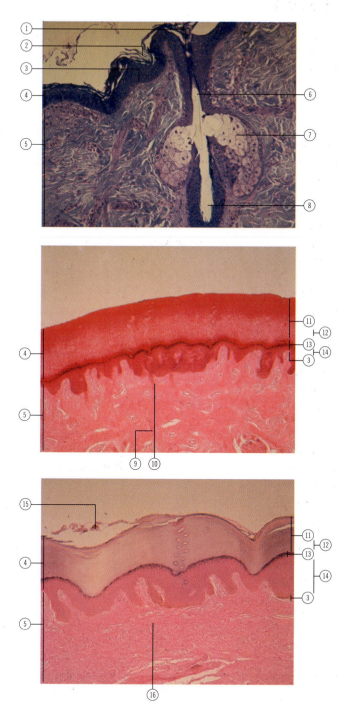

A hair follicle (*top*) in the scalp: a sebaceous gland pushes sebum into the same channel used by the hair bulb as it makes and extrudes a hair. Skin from the fingertip (*middle*) is thick, with a fifth layer, the stratum lucidus. A view (*bottom*) through the thick skin of the sole illustrates dead cells being eroded from the surface.

# THE FULL SKELETON

THE HUMAN SKELETON, THE BODY'S FRAMEWORK, arrived at its present form perhaps five million years ago. By then, it was adapted for a natural upright posture, and had developed a pelvis that was turned upward to centre the upper body directly over the strong lower limbs, and an S-shaped spine supple enough for bending yet stiff enough, with the aid of its musculature, to hold the body erect. In addition to their mechanical functions, the bones store calcium and other minerals with which to make blood cells.

In broad terms, the human skeleton is described as consisting of the axial skeleton (the spine, skull, ribs, and sternum) and the appendicular skeleton (the bones of the limbs and those connecting them to the axial skeleton, such as the pelvic and shoulder-bones).

Altogether, the skeleton usually consists of 206 bones, making up roughly 20 percent of body mass. These are classified generally as long bones (the limbs, clavicles), short bones (the wrists, ankles), flat bones (the sternum, ribs, shoulder blades, cranial bones), or irregular bones (the vertebrae, pelvic and hip-bones, facial bones, and other oddities).

## Key

1. Skull
2. Clavicle
3. Humerus
4. Ulna
5. Pelvic (hip) girdle
6. Femur
7. Patella
8. Tibia
9. Scapula
10. Sternum
11. Rib
12. Vertebral column
13. Radius
14. Fibula

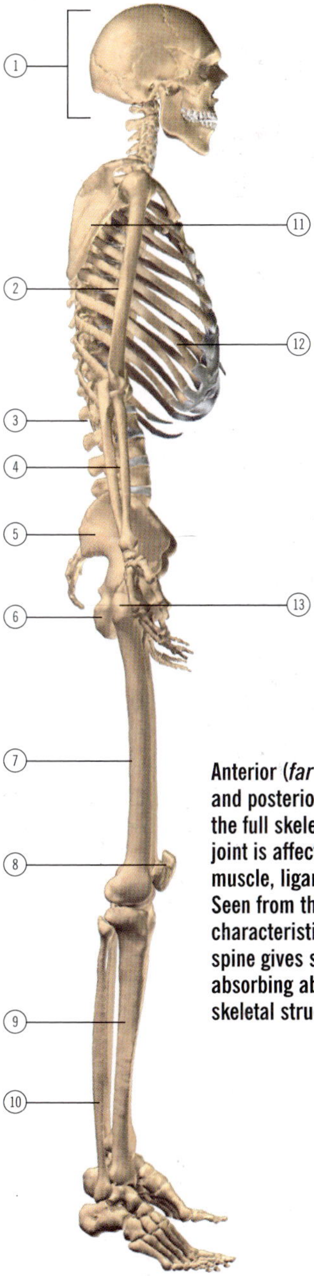

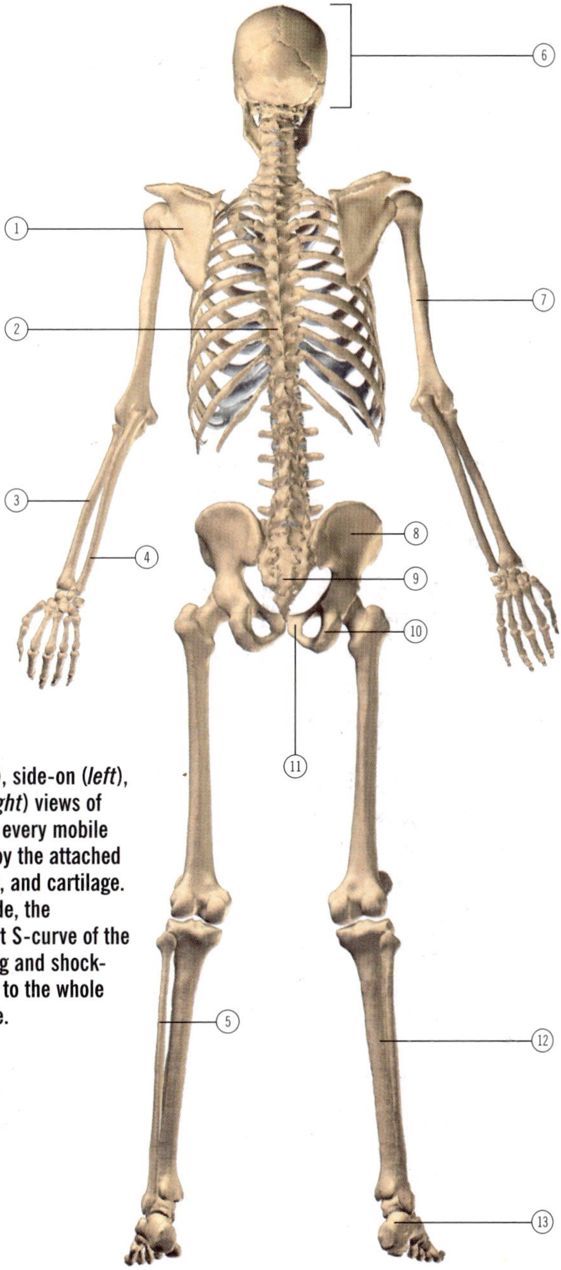

Anterior (*far left*), side-on (*left*), and posterior (*right*) views of the full skeleton: every mobile joint is affected by the attached muscle, ligament, and cartilage. Seen from the side, the characteristic flat S-curve of the spine gives spring and shock-absorbing ability to the whole skeletal structure.

**Key**

| | |
|---|---|
| ① Cranium | ⑧ Patella |
| ② Humerus | ⑨ Tibia |
| ③ Vertebra | ⑩ Fibula |
| ④ Radius | ⑪ Scapula |
| ⑤ Ilium | ⑫ Rib |
| ⑥ Ischium | ⑬ Greater trochanter |
| ⑦ Femur | |

**Key**

| | |
|---|---|
| ① Scapula | ⑧ Ilium |
| ② Vertebra | ⑨ Sacrum |
| ③ Radius | ⑩ Ischium |
| ④ Ulna | ⑪ Pubis |
| ⑤ Fibula | ⑫ Tibia |
| ⑥ Cranium | ⑬ Calcaneus |
| ⑦ Humerus | |

# BONE TYPE AND DEVELOPMENT

BONE IS LIVING TISSUE: WITHIN ITS hard mineralized matrix are living cells that create, destroy, shape, and reshape the bone. The matrix itself serves as storage for minerals, particularly calcium, which is vital to nerve and muscular function and for blood clotting. Blood cells are also made within the bones.

## Bone composition

The bone matrix is composed of protein (about 35 percent, especially **collagen**) and mineral salts (about 65 percent, mainly calcium and phosphate).

Protein gives bone its toughness and some elasticity; minerals provide hardness—it is reckoned that weight-for-weight bone is five times stronger than steel.

These materials combine to form two chief types of osseous (bony) tissue: compact bone and cancellous, or spongy, bone. Compact bone is the stronger of the two, built from tubelike structural units called **osteons**, which have, on average, about six matrix layers from the outside surface to a blood-carrying canal that runs up its centre.

Osteons run lengthwise with the bone and parallel with one another. They surround the bone's inner core and comprise spongy bone and marrow. Cancellous bone comprises a lighter honeycomb lattice of bony struts called **trabeculae**; marrow fills the spaces within this spongy tissue.

Cells called **osteoblasts** manufacture bone. As osteoblasts wall themselves up within the bone matrix, they may become less active **osteocytes**. These maintain the matrix but do not play a part in creating it. A third kind of cells, **osteoclasts**, break down the matrix.

Thus, osteoblasts and osteoclasts are constantly reshaping bones—a process called remodelling—to best meet the stresses applied by muscles or external forces and to store or release calcium, as needed by the body. Osteoblasts are present chiefly in the inside layer of the thin outer membrane, the periosteum, which encases a bone.

## Connective tissue

Closely related to bone in terms of its development and function is cartilage, a type of connective tissue. In common with bone, it arises from specialized cells, young chondroblasts and mature chondrocytes, which form a matrix on a framework of collagen fibres. The resulting tissue, however, is a tough, amorphous, flexible material.

Cartilage develops into three main types, all of which are resilient, elastic, and resistant to compressive and shearing forces. Within the joints it is often present as a smooth, polished surface, which is

## Bone marrow

Bone marrow is a soft, jellylike substance that fills the spaces within a bone—both within its central cavity and in the spongy bone. It comprises:
• Red marrow, which makes blood cells (producing about two million red cells per second). Red marrow is found mainly in flat bones and in the vertebrae, clavicles, pelvis, and the femur's upper end. :
• Yellow marrow, which mostly comprises stored fat and is found in long bones.

lubricated by **synovial** fluid. This cartilage helps minimize wear and tear. Superficially, cartilage also gives shape to some of the body's features, such as the nose and ears.

During the development of the fetus, most bones start out as flexible cartilage, gradually to be replaced, ossified by osteoblasts in a process called endochondral ossification. This process starts before birth and continues through to adolescence.

The skull and a few other bones, including the clavicles, develop from fibrous connective membrane, a transformation termed intramembranous ossification.

In newborn babies the skull is incompletely ossified, which aids the baby's passage down the birth canal and early brain growth; areas of unhardened membrane are called fontanelles. These have usually closed up completely by the age of eighteen months.

A section of human bone (*below*) showing a typical Haversian canal system. The lacunae and canaliculi, the clefts and tubes that suffuse even the densest bone, can clearly be seen.

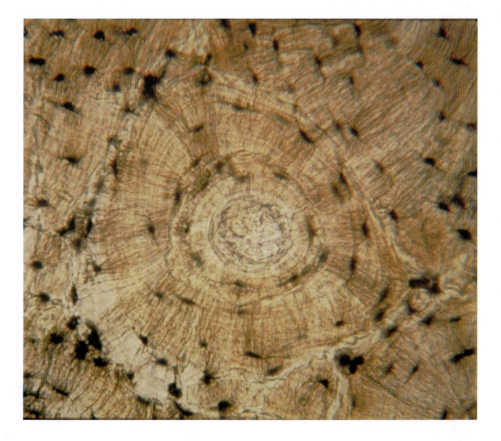

# THE SKULL

THE STRUCTURE OF THE SKULL IS unique: although it consists of 22 bones, only one, the mandible (lower jaw), moves. The rest are closely fitted together at interlocking edges called **sutures**. Of the 22, 8 are cranial bones. These are: at the top, sides, and back the frontal (forehead) and two parietal bones; completing the front, the ethmoid bone; at the lower back and underside of the skull, the occipital bone; at the lower sides, two temporal bones; and forming the centre of the cranial floor, the sphenoid bone. The remaining 14 bones (including the mandible) comprise the facial bones.

Cranial bones house and protect the brain; facial bones provide attachment for the many small muscles of the face and shape the openings for breathing, eating, and vision. Adjoining the nasal passageway are additional hollow spaces, the paranasal sinuses, created by bones in the frontal structures of the head.

There are numerous small holes, called foramina, in the bones of the skull, which accommodate blood vessels and nerves. The largest, through which the spinal cord exits the cranial floor, is the foramen

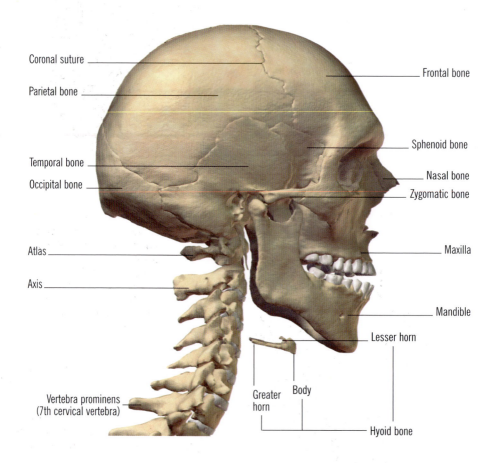

Coronal suture

Parietal bone

Temporal bone

Occipital bone

Atlas

Axis

Vertebra prominens
(7th cervical vertebra)

Frontal bone

Sphenoid bone

Nasal bone

Zygomatic bone

Maxilla

Mandible

Lesser horn

Greater horn

Body

Hyoid bone

magnum. Also at this location can be found the occipital condyle, two knobby projections that articulate with the atlas of the vertebral column to enable the head to nod.

The mandible forms a hinge joint with the temporal bones, which make up the lower side pieces of the cranium. Its motion brings the mandible into exact opposition with the fixed maxilla, the upper jaw. Set into sockets in the borders of each are the 32 teeth, which are not classified as bones.

**Key**
1. Occipital bone
2. Temporal bone
3. Foramen magnum
4. Occipital condyle
5. Vomer
6. Palatine bone
7. Zygomatic bone
8. Maxilla
9. Parietal bone
10. Lambdoidal suture
11. Styloid process
12. Sphenoid bone

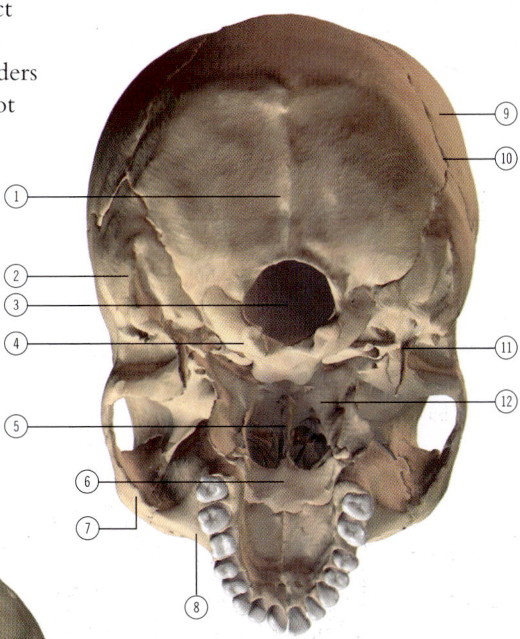

**In frontal (*below*) and lateral (*left*) views, many of the skull's immobile joints are visible. Only the mandible (lower jaw) moves freely. The whole structure is balanced on condyles (rounded, knobby projections) that articulate with the atlas to permit nodding motion of the head.**

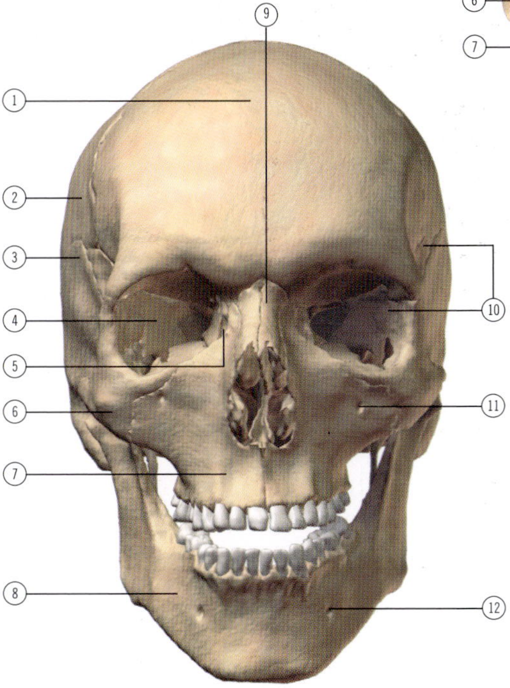

**Seen from below (*above*), the skull's large exit—the foramen magnum—for the spinal cord is flanked by smooth occipital condyles, which fit into ellipsoidal depressions in the atlas. The neck muscles attach to the occipital and temporal bones.**

**Key**
1. Frontal bone
2. Parietal bone
3. Temporal bone
4. Orbit
5. Lacrimal bone
6. Zygomatic bone
7. Maxilla
8. Mandible
9. Nasal bone
10. Sphenoid bone
11. Infraorbital foramen
12. Mental foramen

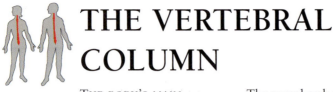

# THE VERTEBRAL COLUMN

THE BODY'S MAIN SUPPORT IS THE vertebral column, also called the spine, spinal column, or backbone. For most of its length, from the skull to the pelvis, it is a structural stack of very similar elements—the vertebrae—which are graduated in size from top (smallest) to bottom and strung together in a long, springy S-shape.

There are 26 vertebrae in all, but the last two, the sacrum and coccyx, have a somewhat different shape, as they are composed of fused vertebrae. The typical vertebra's basic geometry is that of a stubby cylinder (the centrum or body) with a ring (the neural arch) attached at the back. Through the column of rings formed by the long spinal assembly, and protected by it, passes the spinal cord. Weight and strains are borne by the solid cylindrical segments.

The neural arch varies in its details from one vertebra to the next, but consists essentially of two knobby projections emerging from the rear of the vertebral body, which are joined—closing the ring—by a keel-like plate (the spinous process) held between them and extending downward to the next lower vertebra. The inner part of each knob, or process, points slightly upward and articulates with the spinous process of the

**Lateral and anterior views of the vertebral column: the topmost cervical vertebrae, the atlas and axis, form a pivot joint on which the neck rotates. The two bones also form plane joints—analogous to disks in other vertebral joints—between them to either side where their bearing surfaces meet.**

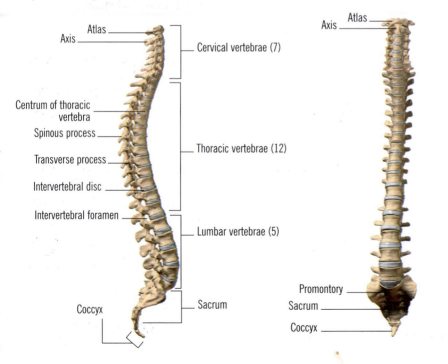

Axis — Atlas — Cervical vertebrae (7)

Centrum of thoracic vertebra
Spinous process
Transverse process
Intervertebral disc
Intervertebral foramen

Thoracic vertebrae (12)

Lumbar vertebrae (5)

Coccyx — Sacrum

Axis — Atlas

Promontory
Sacrum
Coccyx

vertebra above it. The channel created by this closed ring is called the vertebral **foramen**. The outer part, the transverse process, serves as an attachment point for the back muscles and ligaments and, in the thoracic region, for the ribs.

Sandwiched between the vertebral bodies are cartilaginous pads called **intervertebral disks**. These are tough around their circumferences and pulpy toward their centres, and serve to cushion each vertebral joint and transfer weight evenly from one vertebra to the next.

## The vertebrae

Reflecting their position and function, the vertebrae are divided into three groupings: seven small cervical vertebrae that support the neck and allow its flexible movements—the topmost, on which the skull pivots forward and back,

is called the atlas; twelve thoracic vertebrae; and five large lumbar vertebrae, in the small of the back. The sacrum is a special case: formed from five fused bones that make up part of the strong pelvic girdle, it anchors the spine. The last of the vertebrae, the coccyx, is a vestige of the mammalian tail without significant structural importance to the pelvis.

*Clockwise from top left*: cervical vertebra, thoracic vertebra, sacrum, lumbar verterbra. Each is slightly different in shape, but all form a ring at the back, the neural arch, through which the spinal cord passes. The vertebral bodies, or centra, stack atop one another with tough, cartilaginous disks between them. Projections to the side, the transverse processes, provide attachment for the ribs and back muscles.

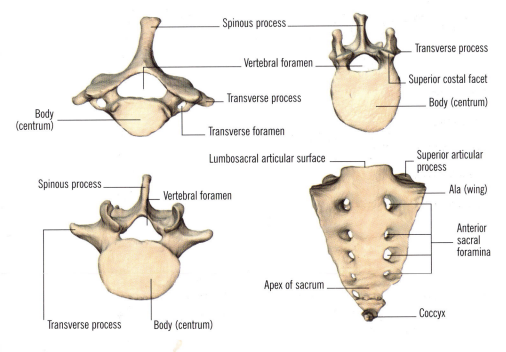

Spinous process

Vertebral foramen

Transverse process

Transverse foramen

Body (centrum)

Transverse process

Superior costal facet

Body (centrum)

Lumbosacral articular surface

Superior articular process

Spinous process

Vertebral foramen

Ala (wing)

Anterior sacral foramina

Apex of sacrum

Transverse process

Body (centrum)

Coccyx

# THE RIBCAGE

THE THORAX (CHEST) IS ENCLOSED BY 12 pairs of ribs, curved flat bones that surround and protect the heart and lungs, as well as most of the upper abdomen and liver. At the back, they are somewhat flexibly attached to the vertebrae (named the thoracic vertebrae) through plane joints, the vertebrocostal joints. From the top, each pair is successively longer in arc than the last, down to the seventh pair—the largest—after which they decrease in size.

Attachment at the front of the ribcage is somewhat freer, to allow regular expansion and contraction of the lungs in breathing. The first seven pairs, the "true" or vertebrosternal ribs, connect through flexible cartilage links to the sternum, or breast-bone, which is flat and bladelike, with notches along its edges where the ribs join. The costal cartilages of rib pairs eight, nine, and ten join with one another and ultimately with the seventh rib's cartilage; these three do not connect directly to the sternum and are called vertebrochondral ribs. Together with pairs eleven and twelve, they are known as "false" ribs. Moreover, pairs eleven and twelve, the "floating" or vertebral ribs, have no link at all to the sternum, and terminate in the abdominal muscles.

The uppermost of the sternum's three parts is the manubrium, which articulates with the clavicles (collar-bones)—a part of the shoulder girdle—and the first pair of ribs. Below the first rib, the manubrium meets the body of the

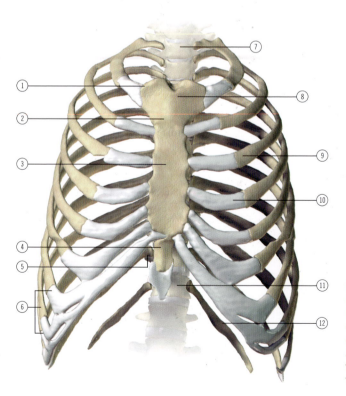

### Key

1. Clavicular notch
2. Sternal angle
3. Body of sternum
4. Xiphoid process of sternum
5. Articulation of rib with vertebra
6. Vertebrochondral ribs
7. 1st thoracic vertebra
8. Manubrium of sternum
9. Vertebrosternal (true) ribs
10. Costal cartilage
11. 12th thoracic vertebra
12. Vertebral (floating) rib

**In an anterior view (*left*), cartilage links between the ribs and sternum are evident. At its wide upper end (the manubrium), just above the first pair of ribs, the clavicles articulate with the sternum.**

sternum at the sternal angle, where there is a cartilaginous joint. The sternal body is thus free to rise and fall during breathing. At the lower end, a flat cartilaginous piece, the xiphoid process, attaches to the thoracic and abdominal muscles. With age, the xiphoid process becomes progressively bonier and less flexible.

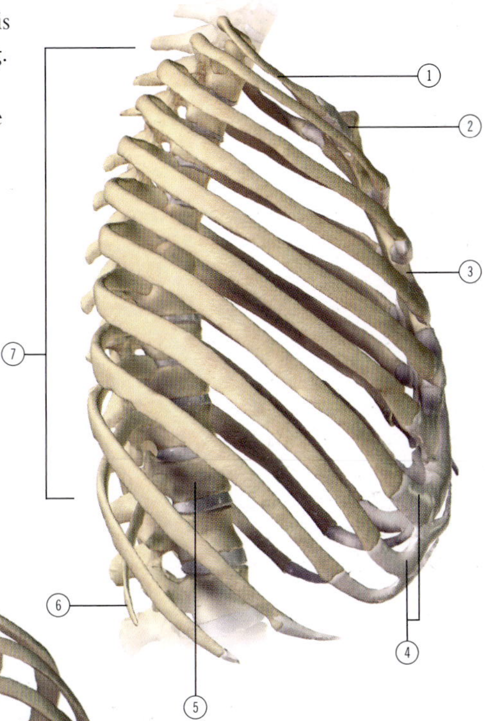

The ribcage in posterior (*below*) and lateral view (*right*). The framework protects the thoracic organs and is flexible enough to permit breathing.

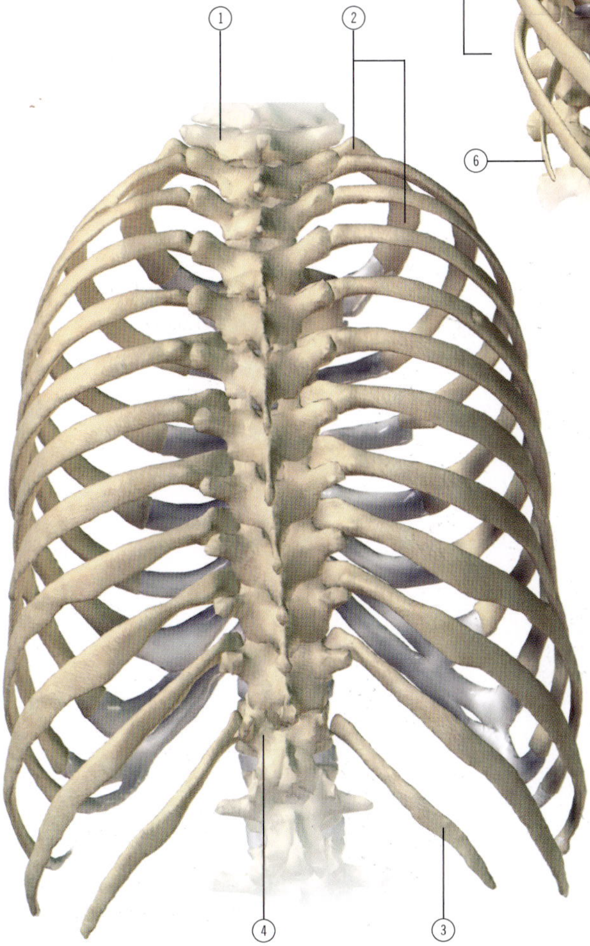

**Key (*top*)**
① First rib
② Manubrium of sternum
③ Sternum
④ Costal cartilage
⑤ 12th thoracic vertebra
⑥ 12th thoracic rib
⑦ Thoracic vertebrae

**Key (*left*)**
① 1st thoracic vertebra
② First rib
③ 12th thoracic rib
④ 12th thoracic vertebra

# THE SHOULDER AND UPPER ARM

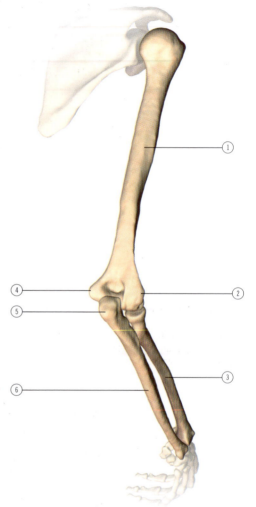

BECAUSE HUMAN BEINGS DO NOT USE their forelimbs for locomotion, like other mammals, the arm has become a highly flexible, adaptable structure. It is attached to the shoulder by a ball-and-socket joint that permits wide rotation of the limb, has a hinge joint at the elbow, and is able to turn itself at the wrist through nearly half a circle.

The shoulder consists of two bones: the clavicle (collar-bone), which connects the shoulder to the rest of the skeletal frame at the sternum; and the scapula (shoulder blade), a triangular bone with a socket, the glenoid fossa, at one of its apexes. The glenoid fossa accommodates the rounded head of the humerus (the upper arm-bone). Anchored to the scapula's large surface are the many muscles of the shoulder, back, and upper arm.

The skeleton of the arm comprises three bones: the humerus, ulna, and radius. The single bone of the upper arm, the humerus, terminates at its **distal** end in a double joint with the two bones of the lower arm: the ulna (inner) and radius (outer). Motion of the ulna is strictly hingelike (in fact, it is held in a groove), though the radius is more freely attached. This allows the radius to twist slightly—it twists relative to the ulna just below the elbow—accounting for the turning motion of the forearm and wrist.

At the distal end, it is the bulging end of the radius that forms the principal part of the wrist joint. Its concave terminal surface, called the styloid process (the ulna has a smaller version of the same thing), articulates with two of the carpal (wrist) bones.

As well as forming joints with the humerus and wrist-bones, the ulna and radius articulate with one another in two places: a notch or groove in the ulna near the elbow, and a similar fitting in the radius, near the wrist. The radius can thus rotate within the upper groove—to which it is confined by a ringlike ligament—while the lower notch rolls on the ulna, twisting the wrist and palm around.

**Key**
1. Humerus
2. Lateral epicondyle
3. Radius
4. Medial epicondyle
5. Olecranon
6. Ulna

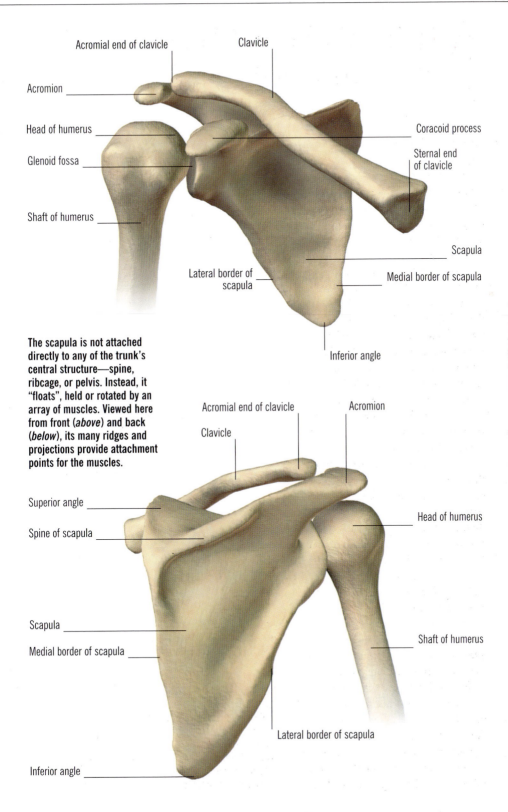

Acromial end of clavicle

Clavicle

Acromion

Head of humerus

Coracoid process

Glenoid fossa

Sternal end of clavicle

Shaft of humerus

Scapula

Lateral border of scapula

Medial border of scapula

Inferior angle

The scapula is not attached directly to any of the trunk's central structure—spine, ribcage, or pelvis. Instead, it "floats", held or rotated by an array of muscles. Viewed here from front (*above*) and back (*below*), its many ridges and projections provide attachment points for the muscles.

Acromial end of clavicle

Acromion

Clavicle

Superior angle

Head of humerus

Spine of scapula

Scapula

Medial border of scapula

Shaft of humerus

Lateral border of scapula

Inferior angle

# THE JOINTS AND LIGAMENTS

WHERE BONES MEET THEY USUALLY FORM a joint, which permits movement in certain directions and allows stability. Immobile joints, such as the **sutures** of the skull, are sometimes referred to as fibrous: that is, their seams are knitted together by cartilage—which often undergoes **ossification** with age. Mobile joints fall into two general classes: synovial and cartilaginous.

Strengthening and stabilizing the joints, attached to the bones, are the ligaments, which are composed of fibrous connective tissue.

Joints that allow relatively free motion (the elbow, shoulder, and knee, etc.) are surrounded by protective cartilaginous capsules, within which the bearing surfaces are glassily smooth and bathed in **synovial fluid**. Less mobile joints, for example, between the vertebrae, lack synovial lubricant and are simply cartilaginous, with pads or disks between the bone surfaces.

The rounded condyles (from word roots meaning "knuckle") at the lower end of the femur rest on cartilaginous wedges, called the medial and lateral meniscus—they are part of the capsule surrounding this synovial joint.

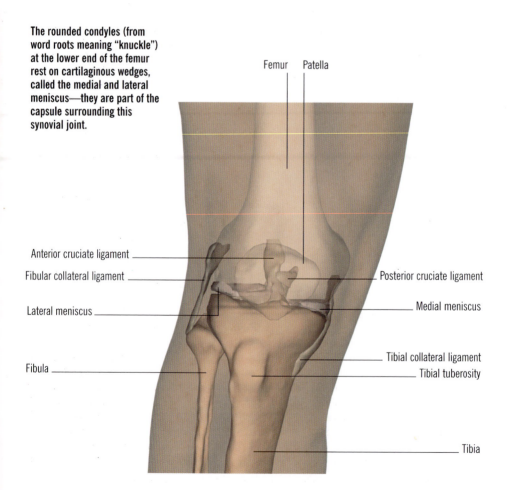

Femur    Patella

Anterior cruciate ligament

Fibular collateral ligament

Lateral meniscus

Fibula

Posterior cruciate ligament

Medial meniscus

Tibial collateral ligament

Tibial tuberosity

Tibia

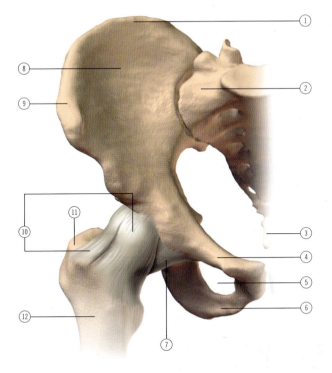

**Key**
1. Iliac crest
2. Sacrum
3. Coccyx
4. Pubis
5. Obturator foramen
6. Ischium
7. Pubofemoral ligament
8. Ilium
9. Anterior superior iliac spine
10. Iliofemoral ligament
11. Greater trochanter
12. Femur

The hip's ball-and-socket joint bears the weight of the trunk above it; although this joint does not have the flexibility of the shoulder, it is more strongly stablized.

## Synovial joints

The freely moveable synovial joints may be broadly classified as:

- ball-and-socket: allows motion in many directions; the rounded end of one bone fits into a rounded cuplike depression in another, e.g., the shoulder or hip.
- hinge: swings in one direction, often with especially strong ligaments to limit the range of motion, e.g., the elbow or knee.
- pivot: works as a swivel, e.g., between the atlas and axis bones of the neck, to permit a wide range of head movements. The body's pivot joints all consist of a central, roughly cylindrical bone surrounded by a ring of ligament and bone. Either of these elements may move: in the case of the atlas and axis, the surrounding ring (of the atlas) moves; in the upper joint between the radius and ulna, the central bone (the radius) rotates within a ring of ligament and bone.
- plane, or gliding, joint: permits short, sliding actions between bones, e.g., within the wrist or ankle (between the carpals or tarsals). Such joints are found between flat or only slightly curved surfaces.
- ellipsoidal, or condyloid, joint: with rocking side-to-side and forward-backward movement, but more limited in one plane than the other, e.g., at the junction of wrist or ankle with the longer limb bones. The fit in a condyloid joint is between an oval cavity in one bone and a matching oval protuberance in the other.
- saddle: also allows movement in two planes, e.g., the thumb joint, at its base. Here, the junction is between a mating cup and knob on each bone.

# THE HAND AND WRIST

THE MOST VERSATILE
PART OF THE skeleton
is the hand, a multiply
jointed structure consisting of 27 bones.

The eight carpal bones (of the wrist)
are short, nugget-like pieces arranged in
two rows of four. **Proximally**—i.e.,
those nearest to the ulna and radius—
are the pisiform (pea-shaped),
triquetrum (three-edged), lunate
(crescent-shaped), and scaphoid (basinlike) bones; **distally**, there are the
hamate (hooked), capitate (round-
headed), and the trapezium and
trapezoid (referring to their regular,
geometrical shapes) bones.

Five longer bones, the metacarpals,
underlie the hand itself and articulate
distally with the 14 phalanges (the
finger-bones).

**Key**
1. Ulna
2. Lunate
3. Triquetral
4. Hamate
5. Metacarpal
6. Proximal
   phalanx
7. Middle phalanx
8. Distal phalanx
9. Radius
10. Scaphoid
11. Trapezoid
12. Trapezium
13. Capitate
14. Proximal phalanx
    of pollex
15. Distal phalanx of
    pollex
16. Pisiform

## The thumb

The thumb's rather special
anatomy positions it
somewhat in front of the
fingers and with a saddle-
shaped depression in its
joint that allows a sweeping
motion across the palm. It
can "oppose" the fingers,
enabling the hand to grasp
and hold objects.

Viewed here palm upward (*right*)
and palm downward (*left*), the
complexity of the wrist joint is
evident. Its seven bones come
together like a piece of repaired
pottery; plane joints between
all the contacting surfaces
permit limited slipping of the
individual parts.

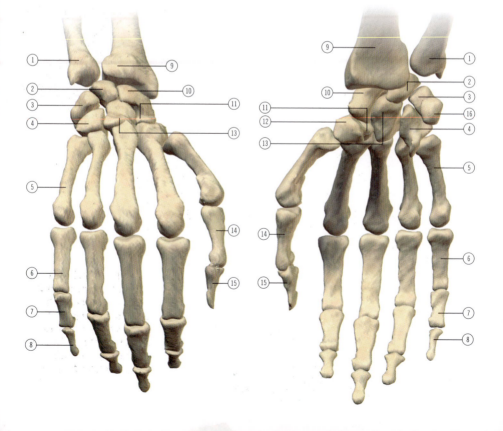

# THE FOOT AND ANKLE

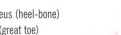

THERE ARE 26 BONES IN THE foot and ankle: 7 tarsal (ankle) bones, 5 metatarsal (sole) bones, and 14 phalanges (the toe-bones).

In the ankle, the talus forms a hinge joint with the tibia's lower end and passes along its weight load to the calcaneus (heel) and to the centrally positioned navicular (boat-shaped) bone. The calcaneus, which hinges on the underside of the talus, has a rearward projection to which the Achilles tendon attaches. The navicular is in contact with the **distal** tarsals, the three cuneiform (wedge-shaped) bones. The remaining tarsal bone, the cuboid, is a one-piece bridge between the calcaneus and the last two metatarsals.

**Key (left)**
1 Fibula
2 Distal tibiofibular joint
3 Lateral malleolus of fibula
4 Tarsals
5 Metatarsals
6 Phalanges
7 Tibia
8 Medial malleolus of tibia
9 Articular surface of medial malleolus
10 Talus
11 Calcaneus (heel-bone)
12 Hallux (great toe)

**Key (right)**
1 Fibula
2 Calcaneus
3 Cuboid
4 Metatarsal of little toe
5 Proximal phalanx
6 Middle phalanx
7 Distal phalanx
8 Tibia
9 Talus
10 Navicular
11 2nd cuneiform
12 3rd cuneiform

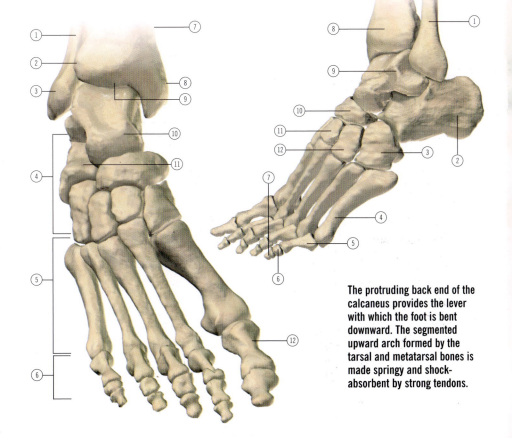

The protruding back end of the calcaneus provides the lever with which the foot is bent downward. The segmented upward arch formed by the tarsal and metatarsal bones is made springy and shock-absorbent by strong tendons.

# THE PELVIS

THE JUNCTION OF THE TORSO AND lower limbs is effected through the pelvis, comprised of two coxal bones (hip-bones), and the sacrum and coccyx, at the base of the spinal column. The coxal bones are each composed of three bones—the ilium, ischium, and pubis—that fuse into one at adolescence. The sacrum and coccyx are formed of fused vertebrae—five for the sacrum and up to five for the coccyx.

**Female pelvis (*top*) and male pelvis (*bottom*), both seen from above (*left*) and below (*right*). To facilitate childbirth, the female pelvis is rounder in its interior outline and wider than the male pelvis.**

**Key (*left*)**
1. Ilium
2. Sacrum
3. Coccyx
4. Iliac tuberosity
5. Iliac crest
6. Greater sciatic notch
7. Ischial tuberosity
8. Pubic symphysis
9. Pubis
10. Ischium
11. Acetabulum
12. Sacral promontory
13. Greater trochanter of femur
14. Inferior pubic ramus
15. Superior pubic ramus
16. Iliopubic eminence
17. Anterior inferior iliac spine

**Key (*right*)**
1. Median sacral crest
2. Articular facet
3. Base of sacrum
4. Sacral promontory
5. Anterior inferior iliac spine
6. Superior pubic ramus
7. Obturator foramen
8. Inferior pubic ramus
9. Pubis
10. Pubic symphysis
11. Anterior superior iliac spine
12. Spine of ischium
13. Greater sciatic notch
14. Iliac crest
15. Ilium
16. Ischium
17. Lateral mass (ala) of sacrum

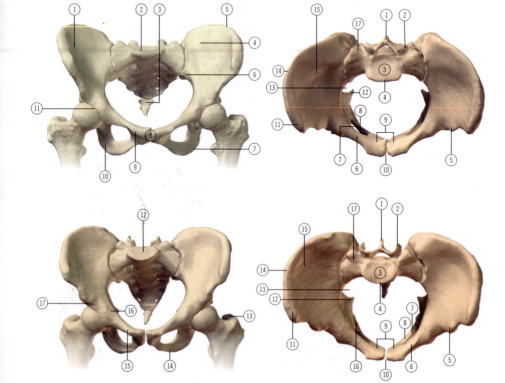

# THE LEG AND KNEE

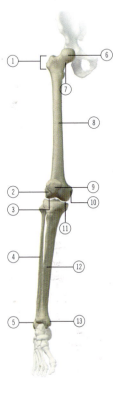

THE LEG-BONES ARE BROADLY SIMILAR to those of the arms, but trade flexibility for stability and strength—the legs must both support the body's weight and carry it in motion. The uppermost leg-bone, the femur (or thigh-bone), is the largest of all the bones and attaches at its head to a socket (the acetabulum) in the side of the pelvis. Just below its head are two small projections, the greater and lesser trochanters, which are attachment sites for thigh and buttock muscles. At the lower end it thickens and splays in knobby processes (condyles) that form the top part of the knee's hinge joint. Shielding that joint at the front is the small triangular patella (kneecap).

The lower leg has two bones: the tibia (shin-bone) and the fibula, a slender bone located to the outside and slightly behind the larger tibia. The tibia's broad, flattened upper surface is a pivot for the femur's condyles, when the knee is flexed. Separating the two bony surfaces, and attached to the tibia, are two extremely tough, smooth cartilage seats (the medial and lateral meniscus) that enable near-frictionless movement in the joint. Controlling and stabilizing the knee are four major ligaments and thirteen supporting muscles.

Lodged under the tibia's head, the fibula carries a portion of the weight transferred at the knee from the femur to the tibia, and thence to the bones of the ankle and foot. Their lower terminus forms the sharp protrusions felt on the outside (fibula) and inside (tibia) of the ankle.

**Key (left)**
1. Greater trochanter
2. Lateral epicondyle
3. Lateral condyle
4. Fibula
5. Lateral malleolus
6. Head of femur
7. Neck of femur
8. Femur
9. Patella
10. Medial epicondyle
11. Medial condyle
12. Tibia
13. Medial malleolus

**The leg's three major bones (left):** the femur's unusual articulation with the tibia, in two condyles, is bound by ligaments and controlled by tendons to confine movement to one plane—as a hinge joint. The hip's ball-and-socket joint (right) allows freer motion.

**Key (below)**
1. Iliac crest
2. Sacrum
3. Coccyx
4. Pubis
5. Obturator foramen
6. Inferior pubic ramus
7. Ischial tuberosity
8. Posterior superior iliac spine
9. Posterior inferior iliac spine
10. Ilium
11. Iliofemoral ligament
12. Ischiofemoral ligament
13. Greater trochanter
14. Femur

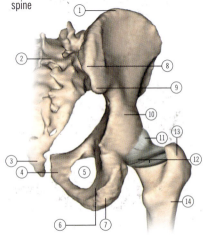

# THE MUSCULAR SYSTEM

THE BODY HAS OVER 640 MUSCLES that move or stabilize some part of the skeleton. We can tense or relax these, consciously, at will. Additionally, internal body systems—digestive, urinary, and reproductive—have their own sets of muscles, but these work without conscious control. The heart, a unique kind of muscle, also has automatic controls. All muscles, however, must have connection to nerves, which bring the signals that enable contraction in the muscle fibres.

Some muscles receive nerve signals from more than one origin along the spinal cord. Or, more accurately, distinct muscle bundles within the same anatomical muscle may be activated (innervated) by different nerve fibres. The brachioradialis (a forearm muscle), for example, connects through fibres running within the radial nerve to impulses that originate in cervical nerves five and six (C5 and C6).

To further complicate matters, few of the body's natural movements are, muscularly speaking, simple affairs. A small gesture, such as raising the arm slightly and rotating the palm outward as if to feel for rain, requires the coordinated action of the shoulder, upper arm, forearm, and palmar muscles—over a dozen in total. Some are active for only part of the exertion, eventually reaching a mechanically neutral point; others merely offer steady resistance to the main movers.

## Key

1. Procerus
2. Zygomaticus minor
3. Zygomaticus major
4. Orbicularis oris
5. Platysma
6. Deltoid
7. Pectoralis major
8. Triceps brachii
9. Biceps brachii
10. Latissimus dorsi
11. Serratus anterior
12. Rectus sheath
13. Pronator teres
14. Brachioradialis
15. Palmaris longus
16. Flexor digitorum superficialis
17. Flexor carpi ulnaris
18. Tensor fasciae latae
19. Levator ani
20. Rectus femoris
21. Ilotibial tract
22. Sartorius
23. Vastus lateralis
24. Vastus medialis
25. Patella
26. Peroneus longus
27. Tibialis anterior
28. Extensor digitorum longus
29. Extensor retinaculum
30. Abductor digiti minimi
31. Abductor hallucis
32. Frontalis
33. Temporalis
34. Orbicularis oculi
35. Levator labii
36. Sternocleidomastoid
37. Infrahyoid
38. Trapezius
39. Pectoralis minor
40. Coracobrachialis
41. Intercostals (anterior)
42. Brachialis
43. External abdominal oblique
44. Supinator
45. Rectus abdominus
46. Flexor pollicis longus
47. Flexor digitorum profundus
48. Internal abdominal oblique
49. Flexor retinaculum
50. Flexor pollicis brevis
51. Abductor digiti minimi
52. Gluteus medius
53. Iliopsoas
54. Pectineus
55. Vastus intermedius
56. Adductor longus
57. Gracilis
58. Gastrocnemius
59. Extensor digitorum longus
60. Extensor hallucis longus
61. Soleus
62. Tibia
63. Dorsal interossei

## Muscle growth

The number of fibres within a muscle does not change much from birth, though the fibres do elongate and thicken during the usual course of human growth and development.

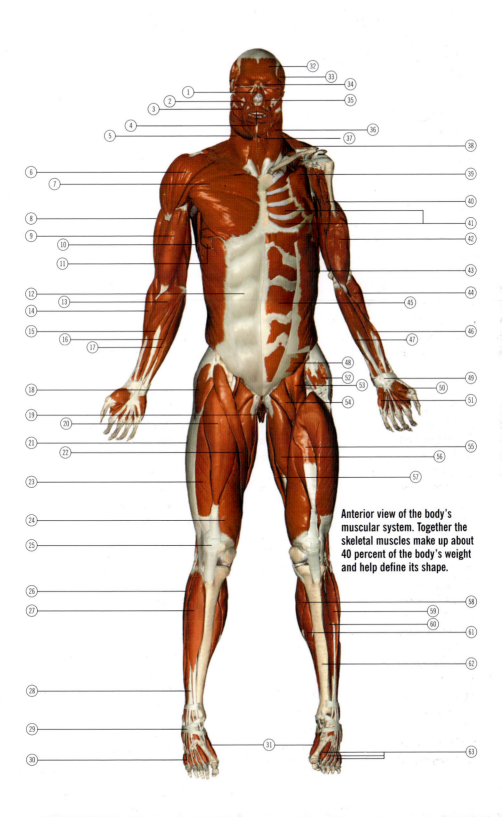

Anterior view of the body's muscular system. Together the skeletal muscles make up about 40 percent of the body's weight and help define its shape.

# THE FULL BODY

THE MUSCLES OF THE BODY MAY be described and classified according to several characteristics, among them their shape, location, or action. Most muscles have names that reflect all or some of this information, using Latin and Greek roots.

## Describing and naming muscles

A muscle is always said to have **origin** and **insertion**: these are its attachment points, usually to skeletal structures, such as the ribs or arm-bones. The origin identifies the more fixed part (or parts) in a muscle's action; insertion is to the part that does most of the moving. If there are several points of origin, a muscle's name may note that fact: the quadriceps femoris, for example, is a muscle arising on the femur (hence femoris) and orginating in four heads (hence quadri + ceps), or segments. Similarly, the biceps brachii and triceps brachii in the arm have, respectively, two and three heads.

Muscle names may also include information about the orientation of a muscle's fibres relative to the midline of the body: "rectus" describes a muscle the fibres of which run parallel to the midline; "transversus" implies that the fibres run in a direction that crosses or is right-angled to the midline; and "obliquus" specifies diagonal (oblique) fibres. When a muscle's fibres run obliquely into its tendon, the muscle is called **pennate** (from a root meaning "feather"). A full feather shape, with diagonal fibres joining a central tendon, is **bipennate**;

with fibres at one side only it is described as **unipennate**. Muscles with a mixture of these junctions, such as the deltoid, are **multipennate**. A circular arrangement of fibres, for example, around the eye, forms a **sphincter**.

The relative shape of a muscle may also be indicated by its name: for example, as with the deltoid (triangular) and trapezius (trapezoid) muscles of the back.

As well as indicating that a muscle is deep-lying or shallow, long or short, muscle nomenclature may reflect other notable qualities, including: large (major, maximus), small (minor, minimus), upper (superior), lower (inferior), inner (internus), outer (externus), front (anterior), and back (posterior).

## Key

1. Semispinalis capitis
2. Sternocleidomastoid
3. Splenius capitis
4. Supraspinatus
5. Infraspinatus
6. Teres minor
7. Rhomboideus major
8. Teres major
9. Triceps brachii
10. Posterior intercostals
11. Flexor carpi ulnaris
12. Supinator
13. Abductor pollicis longus
14. Extensor pollicis longus
15. Dorsal interosseus
16. Gluteus medius
17. Piriformis
18. Adductor minimus
19. Quadratus femoris
20. Vastus lateralis
21. Plantaris
22. Flexor digitorum longus
23. Flexor hallucis longus
24. Galea aponeurotica
25. Epicranius
26. Trapezius
27. Rhomboideus minor
28. Deltoid
29. Triceps brachii
30. Latissimus dorsi
31. External abdominal oblique
32. Anconeus
33. Extensor carpi radialis longus
34. Brachioradialis
35. Extensor carpi radialis brevis
36. Extensor digitorum
37. Extensor carpi ulnaris
38. Extensor digiti minimi
39. Gluteus maximus
40. Levator ani
41. Iliotibial tract
42. Adductor magnus
43. Biceps femoris
44. Semitendinous
45. Semimembranosus
46. Gastrocnemius
47. Soleus
48. Gracilis

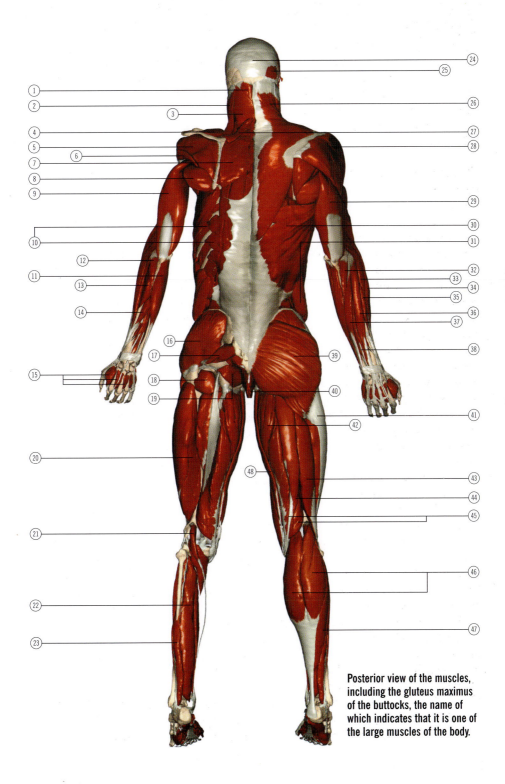

Posterior view of the muscles, including the gluteus maximus of the buttocks, the name of which indicates that it is one of the large muscles of the body.

# TYPES OF MUSCLE

ALL OF THE BODY'S
SKELETAL MUSCLES are
composed of contractile
fibres that together make up striated
muscle—so-called because the muscles
are striped in appearance when viewed
close up. Striated muscle can be activated,
through the nerves, by conscious intent.
Hence it is often also referred to as
"voluntary" muscle.

Another muscle type, smooth muscle,
is found in the internal organs, such as
the intestine. Its fibres are shorter,
unstriped, and arranged in sheets. Its
action is controlled unconsciously, by the
autonomic nervous system, so it is termed
"involuntary" muscle.

Heart muscle is of the first type,
striated, but it is quite different from
other striped muscles as it contracts to its
own unceasing rhythms, normally
without conscious control.

## Muscle structure

The basic units of striated muscle are
**myofibrils**, strands that run the length of
the muscle (up to 12 in/30 cm) and are
gathered together by the thousand to
make individual muscle fibres. Each
myofibril is composed of a string of
linked subsections called **sarcomeres**.
Within each of these are arrays of two
rodlike proteins—actin at the ends and
myosin in the middle. Nerve impulses
cause the two proteins to move ratchet-
like past each other, forcibly shortening
each sarcomere and together shortening

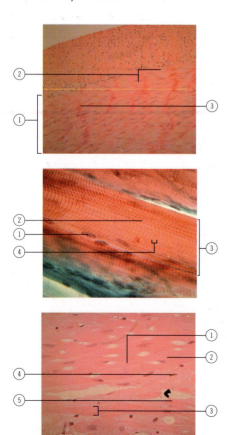

**Key (top)**
① Smooth muscle sheet
② Smooth muscle fibre
③ Nucleus of smooth
   muscle fibre

**Key (middle)**
① Nucleus
② Striation (stripe)
③ Skeletal muscle fibre
④ Sarcomere

**Key (bottom)**
① Striation (stripe)
② Intercalated disc
③ Cardiac muscle fibre
④ Nucleus
⑤ Branch of cardiac
   muscle fibre

**Smooth muscle** (*top*): the
fibres are composed of
short, slightly rounded
filaments aggregating to
form muscular sheets.
**Striated muscle** (*middle*):
uniformly packed
cylindrical filaments are
bundled into long fibres;
the regular arrangement of
its smallest contractile
units, sarcomeres,
produces a banded or
striped appearance.
**Cardiac muscle** (*bottom*):
striped but branched,
cardiac fibres make
junctions with one another
at intercalated disks,
which aid in propagating
electrical impulses.

the entire myofibril. Removing the nerve signal allows the proteins to slide past each other and return to the original configuration.

Muscle fibres are gathered in bundles called **fascicles**; these are held together by connective tissue, **perimysium**, and protectively sheathed by more connective tissue, **epimysium**.

The fibres are not all alike: some have larger available stores of **myoglobin**, a red-coloured protein that holds oxygen. Those with more myoglobin are the "slow-twitch" fibres; they contract more slowly than "fast-twitch" fibres, but tire less easily. White fast-twitch fibres contract quickly—and forcefully—but have low endurance.

A third, intermediate type, red fast-twitch fibres, contract rapidly and have more myoglobin, hence they are slower to fatigue.

Proportions of the fibre types vary from muscle to muscle. A higher fraction of white fast-twitch fibres is found in muscles such as the biceps, for example, because these muscles are used for occasional, strong motions. Intermediate fast-twitch fibres are more numerous in muscles with more need of continual strength, for example, in those used for running. Slow-twitch fibres predominate in muscles that need to maintain activities such as walking, breathing, or holding a posture.

## Tendons

The connective tissue that binds and surrounds the muscles extends past the fleshy "belly" of a muscle, forming dense, flexible cords or sheets (called **aponeuroses**) that may attach one muscle to another or to a bone. These are tendons: bundles of collagen fibres with a white appearance. Where they join to bone, the collagen takes on a specialized form. Called **Sharpey's fibres**, these penetrate into the bone's upper, compact layer, providing firm anchorage. The longer tendons, such as those pulling on the finger joints, run inside sheaths that contain **synovial fluid**, a lubricant.

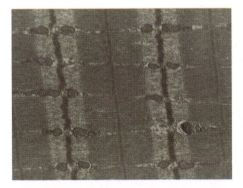

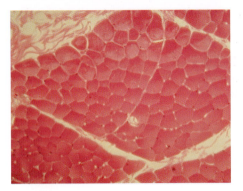

An electron micrograph shows a longitudinal section of skeletal muscle (*top*). Below it, skeletal muscle fibres are seen in cross-section.

# HOW THE MUSCLES WORK

OFTEN, SKELETAL MUSCLES ACT THROUGH LEVERAGE, that is, they cause a bone to turn around a fixed point called the **fulcrum**. The force of the effort, provided by the muscle and acting through a bone, is used to overcome another force, the load of a limb, for example, or an external object. Levers, in elementary physics, are said to be of three kinds: first class, with the fulcrum fixed between effort and load, like a seesaw; second class, where the load is between the fulcrum and effort, like a wheelbarrow; and third class—effort is between the fulcrum and load, a bit like a drawbridge. The majority of levering muscles fall into the third class, pulling on a bone somewhere along its length and pivoting it around a fulcrum, in this case the elbow joint, to move a load, which is the hand and forearm.

In relation to a specific motion, the muscle that causes it is termed an **agonist**. But because muscles work in one direction only, there is usually the need for another muscle to operate in the reverse sense, for example, to return a limb, a finger, or the neck to its original position—an **antagonist**. Muscles that work together to accomplish an action are **synergists**; and muscles that stabilize a bone or joint, so that it becomes a more or less fixed fulcrum, are termed **fixators**. The scapula, when involved in shoulder and arm movement, provides a particularly complex example of how muscles can work together, some holding it in place—as a properly positioned fulcrum—while others raise or lower the arm. At the same time, another group of fixators stabilizes the shoulder joint itself.

It may happen that nothing actually moves, that a muscle works to oppose another muscle or to resist some externally applied force. In other words, a muscle may not actually contract, or be allowed to contract, during its effort. This is called **isometric contraction**. The more straightforward action, in which muscle fibres shorten and thus move a load, is termed **isotonic contraction**.

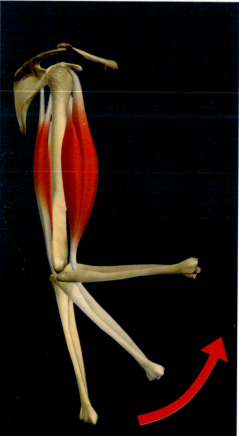

## Muscle action

A muscle's action—which is often reflected in its name—is described in terms of its result:

- flexion: bending; decreases the angle between the parts involved, e.g., bending the arm at the elbow.
- extension: straightening; the opposite of bending, e.g., pulling the thigh into line with the body when rising from a sitting position.
- abduction: movement of a bone away from the body's midline, e.g., raising the arm out to one side.
- adduction: movement towards the midline, e.g., bringing spread fingers back into line.
- elevation: raising, lifting upward, e.g., the mandible (the lower jaw)'s action in closing the jaws.
- depression: downward movement, e.g., the rib's movement as the chest "falls" in expiration.
- supination: turning upward, as to turn something on its "back," e.g., turning the palm up.
- pronation: turning downward, e.g., turning the palm down.
- rotation: turning a bone around its long axis, e.g., the motion of the scapula in bringing the shoulders forward or back.

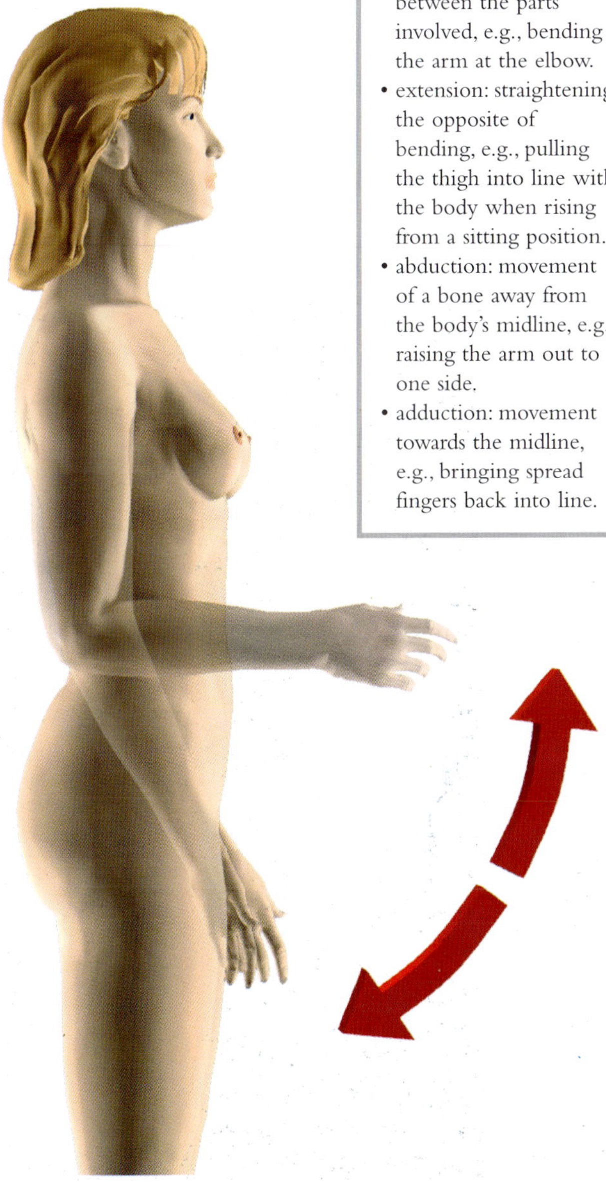

Shown here is the effect of contracting the biceps muscle to raise the lower arm and fist. This is an example of flexion, in which the angle between the upper arm and the low arm decreases.

# THE HEAD AND NECK

THE MUSCLES OF THE FACE AND neck are responsible for pulling the skin into the multitude of contortions that comprise facial expression, as well as controlling movements of the head and jaw. Many insert, wholly or partially, into the skin. While this is unusual, it gives them a direct and shaping effect on these tissues.

## Muscle control

Even more unusual is the fact that the facial muscles are not all controlled in the same way by the brain. Those of the lower face have neural connections chiefly to opposite sides of the brain—in the same way that limbs are directed, contralaterally. That is, the left side of the brain processes movement for the right arm or leg, and vice versa. However, the muscles of the upper face receive input from both sides of the brain, bilateral control, the same as for the trunk and postural muscles. This odd organization appears to arise during embyonic development, when a trunk extension folds itself over the brain, eventually to become the upper face.

## Muscle arrangement

Face muscles are divided into two groups: superficial and deep muscles. The superficial group, which number more than 20 (arranged mostly in left and right pairs), move or stretch part of the face; the deep muscles, of which there are four pairs, are principally involved in chewing action.

The occipitofrontalis muscle has two effects—that is because it has two segments, with widely spaced attachment, but tied into a common **aponeurosis** (tendon). The frontal segment, or venter ("belly"), pulls the skin above the nose upward, wrinkling the forehead and raising the eyebrows; it has insertion into tissue around the eyebrow and at the base of the nose.

With **origins** to the side, on the mastoid process (behind the ear), the occipital venter pulls the scalp backward, an action independent of the frontal venter. Beneath the frontal venter, and blending fibres with it, is the orbicularis oculi. Its three parts surround the eye, moving the skin around it and closing the eyelid.

Muscles that act in the lower face, often imparting facial expression, include: the levator labii superioris, which flares the nostril and turns the lip up; the orbicularis oris, which closes the mouth or purses the lips; the depressor anguli oris, which pulls the corner of the mouth downward; and the depressor labii inferioris, which turns the lower lip outward. There are two zygomatic muscles: zygomaticus major, which draws the angle of the mouth upward and outward as in smiling or laughing; and zygomaticus minor, which elevates the upper lip, exposing the maxillary teeth. The buccinator inserts into the orbicularus oris and acts to press the cheeks against the teeth, as in whistling.

The platysma, a larger muscle that arises in the shoulder and sheaths the front of the neck, can contribute to facial expression, opening the mouth (acting on the mandible, the lower jaw) or pulling the angle of the mouth downward. It is also able to lift and tighten the skin of the neck and chest.

**The muscles that create facial expression often have direct insertion into skin tissue, giving them visible, finely differentiated play in the face.**

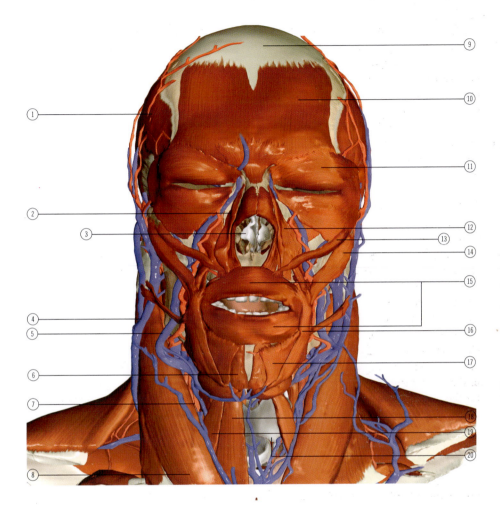

**Key**

1. Temporalis
2. Levator labii superioris alaeque nasi
3. Nasal cartilage
4. External jugular vein
5. Facial vein
6. Mentalis
7. External carotid artery
8. Sternocleidomastoid
9. Galea aponeurotica
10. Frontalis
11. Orbicularis oculi
12. Levator labii superioris
13. Zygomaticus minor
14. Zygomaticus major
15. Orbicularis oris
16. Depressor anguli oris
17. Depressor labii inferioris
18. Sternohyoid
19. Omohyoid
20. Larynx

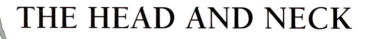

# THE HEAD AND NECK

LOCATED SLIGHTLY TO THE SIDE OF the face are several more expressive muscles: the risorius, which widens the mouth, pulling the corner **laterally**; the zygomaticus major, which raises the mouth corners; and the buccinator, which flattens the cheeks, drawing them inward as, for example, to suck through a straw.

Two strong muscles, the masseter and temporalis, move the lower jaw and power the action of chewing. The masseter, the lower of the two, arises from the maxilla and zygomatic arch; the temporalis originates at the hollow of the temple. Both are inserted in several places onto the mandible and have similar actions: elevating the mandible (closing the jaws) and assisting in motion from side to side and outward and inward.

Two other pairs of muscles, the pterygoids, help control and stabilize the action of the larger sets. The medial pterygoids assist in masseter action, closing the jaw forcefully, but also act with the lateral pterygoids to adjust the position of the mandible, giving it side-to-side mobility or causing it to jut forward. Thus, the teeth are brought together in an efficient overlap, or "bite".

A strap of muscle running up either side of the neck connects the shoulder and skull, and can rotate the head to one side or the other. These head-turning muscles are the sternomastoids (full name sternocleidomastoideus); they arise on each clavicle and have insertion at the mastoid process. When acting together, they flex the head, bending it forward—and thus opposing the trapezius, which pulls the head and shoulders backward.

The stronger muscles of the head and neck are seen here in side view: these are the masseter, temporalis, sternocleidomastoid, and trapezius. The first two close the jaw during chewing; the other two hold and position the head.

**Key**
1. Frontalis
2. Orbicularis oculi
3. Procerus
4. Nasalis
5. Facial vein
6. Zygomaticus
7. Orbicularis oris
8. Buccinator
9. Masseter
10. Depressor angularis oris and labii inferioris
11. Submandibular gland
12. Digastric (anterior)
13. Sternohyoid
14. Omohyoid
15. External jugular vein
16. Clavicle
17. Galea aponeurotica
18. Temporalis
19. Occipitalis
20. Superficial temporal vein
21. Occipitalis vein
22. Parotid gland
23. Trapezius
24. Sternocleidomastoid

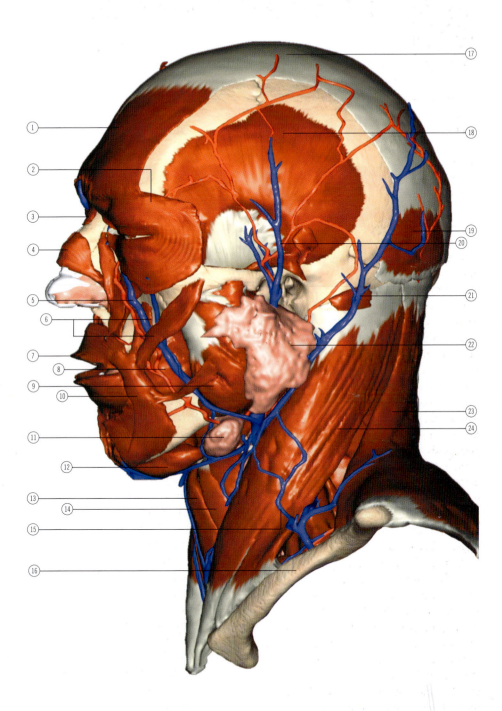

# THE THORAX

THE MUSCLES OF THE THORAX ARE mostly broad and flat, lying on top of and across one another in layers upon the underlying skeletal structures of the thoracic cavity. Principally, the thoracic muscles control breathing and movement of the arm and shoulder. One of the thoracic muscles, the trapezius, also helps move the head.

Those pulling on the scapula or ribs, but not involved in arm motion, include the serratus anterior, the rhomboids major and minor, the trapezius, the pectoralis minor, and the many pairs of intercostal muscles. With the exception of the trapezius, these are all deep muscles, overlain by superior thoracic muscles—the pectoralis major, a large fan-shaped muscle, and the latissimus dorsi.

The serratus anterior **originates** in the upper eight or nine ribs and inserts at the scapula (shoulder blade), which it pulls forward and down, as well as helping to rotate it, particularly in raising the arm above shoulder level. (The serratus posterior muscles, both superior and inferior, respectively elevate and depress the ribs. Their attachments are at the vertebrae and ribs, in the back.)

Assisting the serratus anterior in its actions is the pectoralis minor muscle,

which also arises in the upper ribs and is inserted onto the scapula, near the coracoid process.

The trapezius is an extensive muscle—superficially covering the back and shoulder like a shawl; it arises from attachments to all of the thoracic vertebrae, plus the 7th cervical, and inserts at the clavicle (collar-bone) and two points on the scapula. It elevates and retracts (pulls backward) the scapula, and assists in rotating it, and also helps support and extend the head.

Acting in a similar way on the scapula, and lying underneath the trapezius, are the rhomboid major and, above it, the rhomboid minor. These two muscles also originate at the vertebrae—the rhomboid major at the 2nd to 5th thoracic; the rhomboid minor at the 7th cervical and 1st thoracic—and insert on the scapula.

The intercostal muscles connect adjacent ribs. There are 44 in all: 11 pairs of external intercostals, which elevate the ribs during inspiration, and 11 pairs of internal intercostals, which depress the ribs and may assist in expiration. The internal muscles arise in cartilage of the rib above; the external muscles arise on the rib's border. Both insert in the rib border below.

**Key**

1. Platysma
2. Deltoid
3. Pectoralis major
4. Latissimus dorsi
5. Serratus anterior
6. Rectus sheath
7. Omohyoid
8. Sternocleidomastoid
9. Sternohyoid
10. Trapezius
11. Pectoralis minor
12. Coracobrachialis
13. Intercostals (anterior)
14. Brachialis

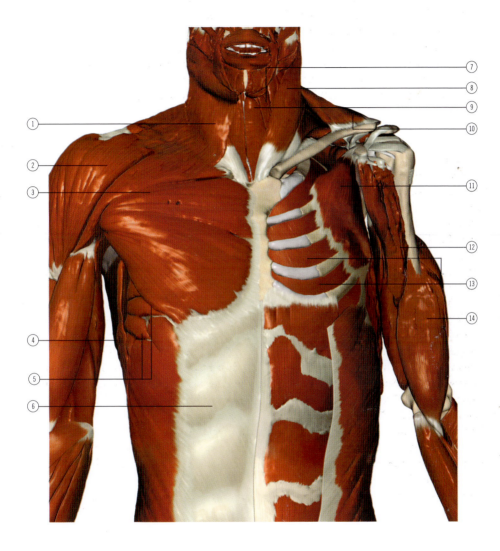

1
2
3
4
5
6
7
8
9
10
11
12
13
14

The deeper-lying thoracic
muscles position and hold the
scapula or control respiration.
The superficial muscles have
several actions, assisting in
movement of the arm or head,
or in forced inspiration.

# THE SHOULDER AND CHEST

THE SHOULDER IS THE BODY'S MOST flexible joint, which is why it is also somewhat unstable. To control its wide range of motion and hold it together, the joint is wholly clad in muscle (nine muscles in total cross the shoulder joint), some of which provide anchoring to the sternum (the breast-bone) and vertebrae, others to the clavicle (the collar-bone) and broad scapula (the shoulder blade) that form the shoulder girdle.

The chief movers of the arm are the deltoid, pectoralis major, teres major, and latissimus dorsi muscles, but several others assist in scapula movement and joint stability, including the serratus anterior, rhomboids major and minor, and the trapezius—the muscles of the thorax.

Describing shoulder movement can be confusing: flexing refers to arm-lifting motions to the front, extension is downward and back; abduction brings the arm up and out to the side, adduction returns it to the body's side; rotation (of the whole arm, not just the forearm) is lateral when turning out, medial when turning in. Many of the arm's natural motions are, of course, compounds of several basic muscular actions.

Four muscles mainly provide shoulder joint stability; together they are often called the **rotator cuff muscles**: the infraspinatus, supraspinatus, subscapularis, and teres minor. All **originate** on the scapula and **insert** at the humerus. Their tendons connect with the fibrous capsule that envelops the shoulder joint.

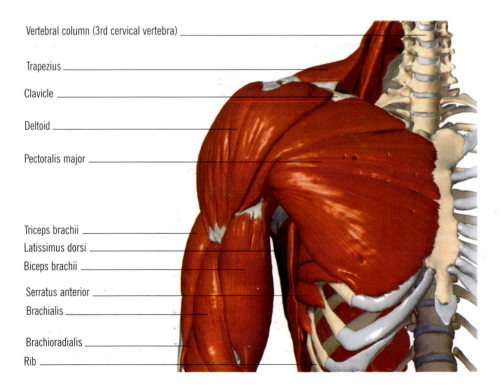

Vertebral column (3rd cervical vertebra)

Trapezius

Clavicle

Deltoid

Pectoralis major

Triceps brachii

Latissimus dorsi

Biceps brachii

Serratus anterior

Brachialis

Brachioradialis

Rib

Most prominent in arm movement is the deltoid, which originates both at the scapula and clavicle and is inserted in the humerus. Its anterior fibres participate in flexing the arm and medial rotation; the posterior fibres act in extending the arm and lateral rotation. All of its fibres, however, take part in its principal action, which is to abduct the arm.

The other important shoulder muscles all act as arm **adductors**, **antagonists** in this sense to the deltoid. The pectoralis major, which originates at the sternum, rib cartilages, and clavicle, and inserts to the humerus, covers the fleshy upper area of the chest. It adducts, flexes, and medially rotates the arm. A smaller scapular muscle, the corachobrachialis, also adducts and flexes. A posterior muscle, the latissimus dorsi, adducts and powerfully extends the arm and medially rotates it.

It is a broad sheet of muscle, covering much of the lower back, originating in the lower vertebrae and iliac region of the pelvis, and inserting on the humerus. The teres major, located under the joint, adducts, extends, and laterally rotates the arm. It is another of the seven shoulder muscles that originate on the scapula, but its insertion is in the humerus.

The "lats" and "pecs", with their wide thoracic attachment, also help adjust trunk posture. The pectoralis lifts the chest, too, in forced inspiration (intake of breath).

**Posterior and anterior views of the shoulder: Superficially, the deltoid gives the shoulder its rounded fleshy shape; it is also the prime mover in arm abduction. Lying deep to the deltoid are many muscles that oppose or assist it in arm movement, and some that hold the shoulder joint in place.**

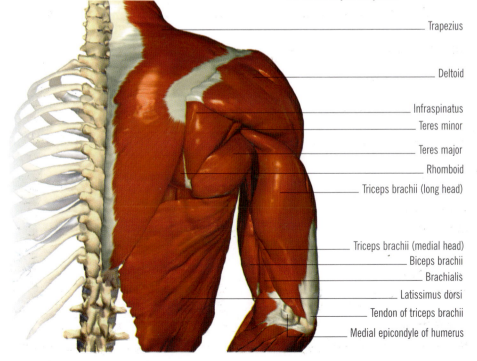

Trapezius
Deltoid
Infraspinatus
Teres minor
Teres major
Rhomboid
Triceps brachii (long head)
Triceps brachii (medial head)
Biceps brachii
Brachialis
Latissimus dorsi
Tendon of triceps brachii
Medial epicondyle of humerus

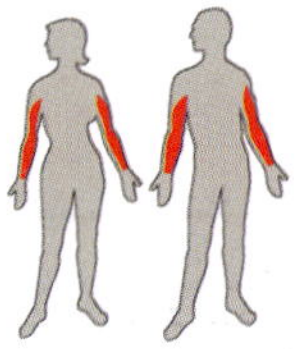

# THE BICEPS BRACHII

THE UPPER ARM MUSCLES INCLUDE THREE that flex the forearm—the biceps brachii, brachialis, and brachioradialis—and one antagonist that extends it, the triceps brachii. The biceps, so-called because it divides into two "heads", arises from the coracoid process of the scapula and from a tubercle (nodule) above the shoulder socket (the glenoid fossa); it inserts into the radius.

**Key (*below*)**

① Deltoid
② Scapula
③ Teres minor
④ Teres major
⑤ Triceps brachii
⑥ Brachialis
⑦ Extensor carpi radialis longus
⑧ Lateral epicondyle of humerus
⑨ Extensor carpi radialis brevis
⑩ Extensor digitorum
⑪ Extensor carpi ulnaris
⑫ Medial epicondyle of humerus
⑬ Olecranon of ulna
⑭ Anconeus

**Posterior view of the right shoulder (*right*) and lateral view of the right shoulder and upper arm (*bottom*): the triceps is strongly inserted at the elbow, into the ulna, which it levers into extended position. Opposing it in action are the biceps, brachialis, and brachioradialis.**

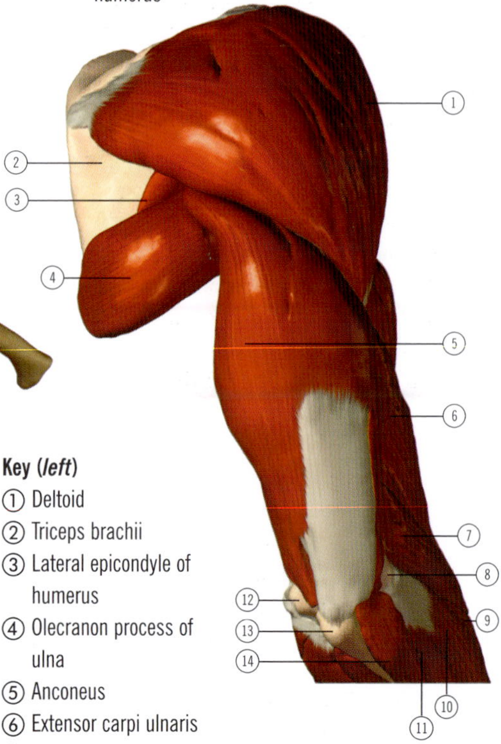

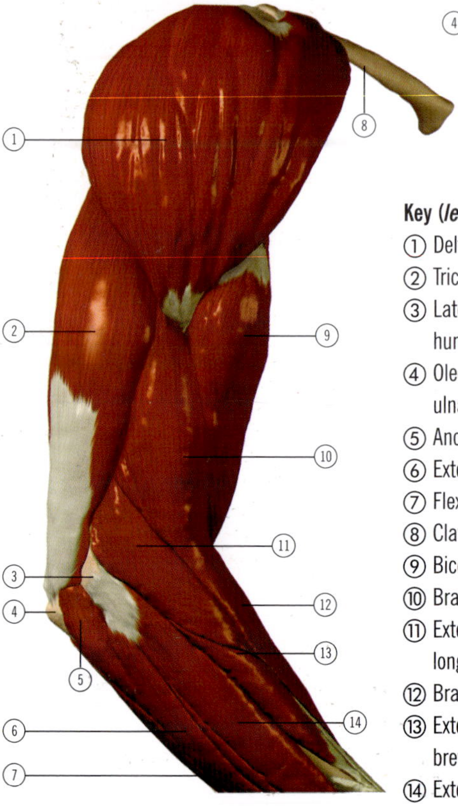

**Key (*left*)**

① Deltoid
② Triceps brachii
③ Lateral epicondyle of humerus
④ Olecranon process of ulna
⑤ Anconeus
⑥ Extensor carpi ulnaris
⑦ Flexor carpi ulnaris
⑧ Clavicle
⑨ Biceps brachii
⑩ Brachialis
⑪ Extensor carpi radialis longus
⑫ Brachioradialis
⑬ Extensor carpi radialis brevis
⑭ Extensor digitorum

The biceps also enables the forearm to twist so that the wrist and palm turn upward—as if laying the forearm on its "back", that is, supine. Acting jointly with the biceps to flex the forearm, but through a shorter connection, is the brachialis; it originates in the lower half of the humerus and is inserted onto a projection (a tubercle) of the ulna.

The brachioradialis, originating on the lower humerus and inserted into the lower radius, aids in flexing the forearm and in pronating it: **pronation** is the opposite of supination; in this case turning the wrist and palm downward.

A three-headed muscle, the triceps brachii, arises from two attachment points on the humerus and one at the scapula, in the glenoid region. It is inserted at the knobby upper surface of the ulna's head, called the olecranon. The whole muscle acts to extend the forearm, but its longest head—at the scapula—also helps extend the arm out to one side (**abduction**).

**Key**
1. Head of humerus
2. Deltoid
3. Coracobrachialis
4. Biceps brachii
5. Brachioradialis
6. Extensor carpi radialis longus
7. Flexor carpi radialis longus
8. Tendon long head triceps (cut)
9. Subscapularis
10. Triceps brachii
11. Medial head triceps
12. Brachialis
13. Pronator teres
14. Palmaris longus
15. Flexor carpi ulnaris

Medial view of the shoulder and arm showing the biceps brachii. The upper arm has been disarticulated to expose the head of the humerus. The pectoralis major and a portion of the deltoid muscle have been removed, bringing the long head of the triceps into full view.

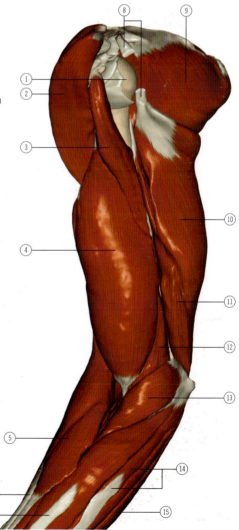

# THE FOREARM AND HAND

MOST OF THE MUSCLES THAT MOVE the wrist and fingers are in the forearm; smaller muscles in the hand refine finger and thumb motion. Forearm muscles originate at the elbow and reach their insertions, at the wrist or finger-bones, via long tendons running inside lubricating **synovial** sheaths. The tendons are held in place at the wrist by bracelet-like fibrous bands called **retinacula**.

The anterior (inner) forearm muscles are mostly flexors: the flexor digitorum superficialis bends the fingers; the flexor carpi ulnaris, flexor carpi radialis, and palmaris longus all flex the wrist. The flexor carpi ulnaris also adducts the hand,

while the flexor carpi radialis abducts it: these are the sideways motions of the hand at the wrist—adduction pulls it back into line with the forearm, abduction moves it outward. The palmaris longus tenses the hand, tightening the palmar aponeurosis. The flexor pollicis longus, another anterior muscle, flexes the thumb. The pronator teres twists the forearm, **pronating** it, so that the wrist and palm

The forearm and hand, seen palm up (*left*) and palm down (*right*): the larger hand muscles are located in the forearm, exerting force through sheathed tendons.

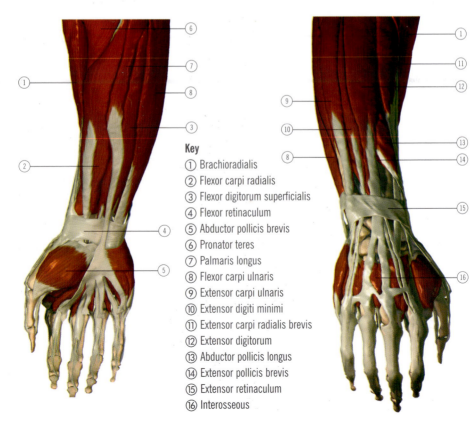

**Key**
1. Brachioradialis
2. Flexor carpi radialis
3. Flexor digitorum superficialis
4. Flexor retinaculum
5. Abductor pollicis brevis
6. Pronator teres
7. Palmaris longus
8. Flexor carpi ulnaris
9. Extensor carpi ulnaris
10. Extensor digiti minimi
11. Extensor carpi radialis brevis
12. Extensor digitorum
13. Abductor pollicis longus
14. Extensor pollicis brevis
15. Extensor retinaculum
16. Interosseous

are made to turn downward. And the brachioradialis has several actions, principally assisting the biceps brachii to flex the forearm, but also aiding in pronation and extension of the forearm.

The **posterior** (outer side) muscles of the forearm are mostly extensors, **antagonists** to the flexors. They include the extensors carpi radialis longus and brevis (extend the wrist and abduct the hand), the extensor carpi ulnaris (extends the wrist and adducts the hand), the extensor digitorum (extends the fingers), the extensors pollicis brevis and longus (extend the thumb), and the extensor digiti minimi (extends the little finger).

There are smaller muscles within the hand that assist in finger movements, making them more precise and controlled. Among them are the thenar muscles, including the flexor pollicis brevis and abductor pollicis brevis (flex or abduct the thumb); and the opponens pollicis (medially rotates the thumb). There are also the interosseus and lumbrical ("wormlike") muscles between the metacarpals (which flex the knuckles but extend the fingers).

**The hand, palm up: four string-like lumbricales muscles assist in flexing the fingers at the first joint and in straightening the distal two joints. Overlying these deeper muscles and tendons, and tying together their borders and sheaths, is the palmar aponeurosis.**

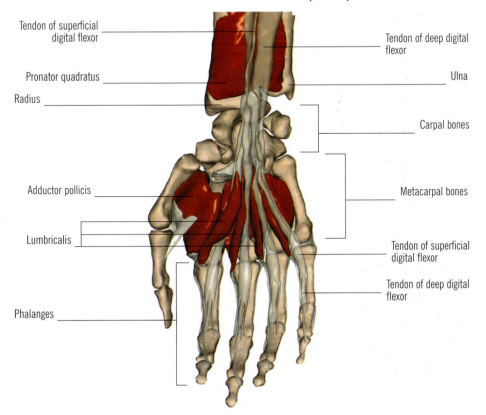

Tendon of superficial digital flexor

Pronator quadratus

Radius

Adductor pollicis

Lumbricalis

Phalanges

Tendon of deep digital flexor

Ulna

Carpal bones

Metacarpal bones

Tendon of superficial digital flexor

Tendon of deep digital flexor

# THE ABDOMEN

THE ABDOMINAL WALL
IS A GROUP of four
symmetric, flat muscles
and their straplike connective tendons,
which support and confine the abdominal
organs. These muscles assist in trunk
rotation and forward or sideways flexing;
they resist any tendency of the muscles in
the back to pull too far in that direction.

In the front and centre is the rectus
abdominus, originating from the pubic
bone and inserted into rib cartilages and
the xiphoid process (at the **distal** end of
the sternum). It **originates** in part, as
well, at the lower end of the linea alba, a
flat band of tendon formed at the central
junction of the other three abdominal

**Key**

1. Rectus sheath
2. Tensor fasciae latae
3. Rectus femoris
4. Levator ani
5. External abdominal
   oblique
6. Rectus abdominus
7. Internal abdominal
   oblique
8. Gluteus medius
9. Iliopsoas
10. Pectineus

**Anterior view of the abdomen:
the rectus sheath is a two-
layered fibrous sheet that
covers the abdomen and
surrounding segments of
the rectus abdominus; its
layers fuse at the midline to
form a long tendonlike band,
the linea alba.**

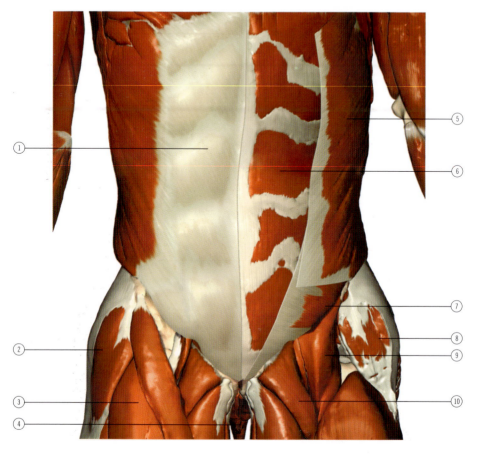

muscles: the external oblique, internal oblique, and transversus abdominus.

The external oblique, at either side of the rectus abdominus, arises in the lower ribs and is inserted by a wide aponeurosis into the pelvic girdle. Its fibres run down, in towards the midline. Underneath is the internal oblique, originating in the posterior pelvis and inserted onto the lower ribs. Its fibres run at right angles to those of the external oblique. Below this is the transversus abdominus, whose fibres run horizontally across the abdomen, and which originates in the pelvic girdle and from the inside surfaces of the lower rib cartilages. It inserts at the upper and lower parts of the linea alba and into the pubis.

**Key**

1. Posterior intercostals
2. Gluteus medius
3. Piriformis
4. Quadratus femoris
5. Adductor minimus
6. External abdominal oblique
7. Gluteus maximus
8. Levator ani

**The abdomen, posterior view (lumbar region of the back): three layers of lumbar fascia— the lumbar aponeurosis— originate in attachments at the spine. These fuse together to form one sheet, which serves as partial origin for the transversus abdominis and internal oblique.**

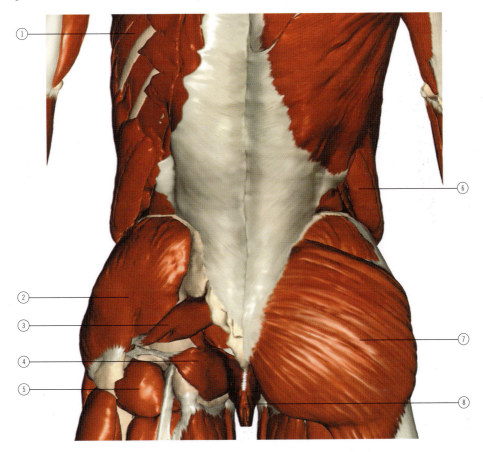

# THE PELVIS, THIGH, AND KNEE

THE HIP AND UPPER LEG ARE moved by the body's most powerful muscles; they accomplish all the flexing, straightening, and rotating movements necessary for locomotion and collectively help maintain balance.

Anterior thigh muscles flex the hip (lift the thigh), rotate and adduct the leg (bring it inward), and extend the knee (straighten it). Posterior thigh and hip muscles include the gluteus maximus; they extend the hip, straightening it by pulling on the thigh from behind, rotate and abduct the leg (move it outward to the side), and flex it at the knee.

## The anterior muscles

Of the anterior muscles, the quadriceps femoris is the largest; indeed, it is a bundle of four muscles—the rectus femoris, vastus lateralis, vastus medialis, and vastus intermedius—that are joined by their insertion in common into tendons that attach to the tibia and patella. The quadriceps is thus said to have four heads, which **originate** in various attachment points in the pelvic girdle and upper femur.

The thigh has five adductor muscles, all arising in the pelvic region of the pubis: the pectineus, gracilis, adductor brevis, adductor longus, and adductor magnus. All but the gracilis insert directly, or through connective bands, into the femur; the gracilis (and sartorius) inserts at the upper end of the tibia. The adductors also rotate the thigh and, with the pectineus and sartorius, may assist in flexing it.

The gracilis and sartorius flex the leg, but the long ribbonlike sartorius (the

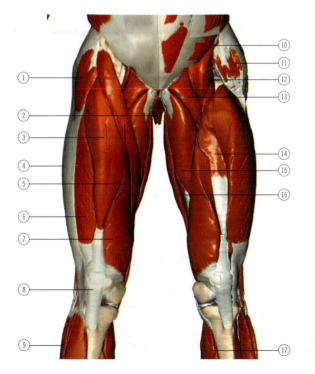

### Key
1. Tensor fasciae latae
2. Levator ani
3. Rectus femoris
4. Iliotibial tract
5. Sartorius
6. Vastus lateralis
7. Vastus medialis
8. Patella
9. Peroneus longus
10. Internal abdominal oblique
11. Gluteus medius
12. Iliopsoas
13. Pectineus
14. Vastus intermedius
15. Adductor longus
16. Gracilis
17. Gastrocnemius

**The anterior thigh is mostly overlain by the four masses of the large quadriceps femoris.**

"tailor's muscle") also rotates the tibia medially when the knee is bent. The sartorius and tensor fasciae latae originate in the pelvic girdle, the ilium; both insert in the tibia, though the tensor muscle is connected by the iliotibial tract. The tensor fasciae extends and laterally rotates the leg (but if the foot is off the ground, it assists in medial rotation of the thigh).

Neither truly **anterior** nor **posterior**, but agreeing with the anterior group in action, are two powerful muscles, the psoas major and iliacus. They flex the thigh but also pull the pelvis and trunk up when the thigh is fixed or restrained. Arising in attachments to the lumbar vertebrae, the ilium and sacrum, they insert by a common tendon into the proximal femur and are usually considered one compound muscle, the iliopsoas. The psoas major also medially rotates the free leg.

# The posterior muscles

The gluteus maximus originates in multiple attachment points in the pelvic girdle and has insertion in the femur and iliotibial tract, which attaches to the tibia. It extends and laterally rotates the thigh, and helps stabilize the knee. Although used along with other muscles in walking, its strongest action is to provide powerful hip extension in activities such as running or climbing stairs.

Other muscles in this group, the gluteus medius and gluteus minimus, also attached at the pelvis and femur, act similarly in their posterior fibres, but the anterior fibres of both these muscles flex the thigh and rotate it medially; they have a steadying effect on the pelvis when walking. Together these three muscles comprise most of the buttock. All of them abduct the thigh.

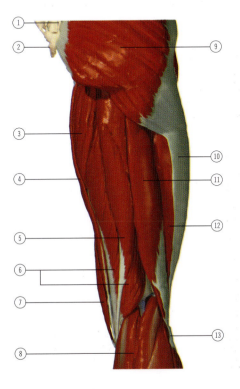

**Key**

① Sacrum
② Coccyx
③ Adductor magnus
④ Gracilis
⑤ Semitendinosus
⑥ Semimembranosus
⑦ Sartorius
⑧ Gastrocnemius
⑨ Gluteus maximus
⑩ Iliotibial tract
⑪ Biceps femoris
⑫ Vastus lateralis
⑬ Tendon of biceps femoris

The posterior muscles of the thigh include the body's largest, the gluteus maximus; they straighten the hip or bend the knee, and abduct the thigh. The hamstrings (the biceps femoris, semimembranosis, and semitendinosis) do most of the work in walking, and run in parallel down the back side of the thigh; the gluteus finds attachment to the tibia via the iliotibial tract, a thick fibrous band extending the length of the thigh, along its outer side.

# THE LEG AND FOOT

THE ACTION OF THE FOOT IN walking is principally to provide extra push as the foot leaves the ground. The foot muscles that power this motion, **plantar flexion** (extension to straighten the toes), are the strongest. **Dorsiflexion** (bending the foot upward) is more useful in balance and stability—and in keeping the foot from dragging. These muscles are not as substantial as those used in plantar flexion. The muscles of the foot also maintain a springy arch, flex or extend the toes, or turn the sole up to one side or the other. A muscle is said to **invert** the sole if it turns inward, to **evert** if it turns outward.

Running along the **posterior** of the lower leg are the gastrocnemius and soleus, the chief muscles of plantar flexion. Both are inserted into the heel-bone (calcaneus) via the calcaneal (Achilles) tendon. Another pair of plantar flexors, the peroneus brevis and peroneus longus, run laterally (on the outside) and are inserted onto the fifth metatarsal bone. They also evert the foot, helping to keep it flat on the ground. Two anterior muscles, the flexor digitorum longus and flexor hallucis longus, also plantar flex the foot: the first flexes the small toes, too, and the second flexes the big toe (hallux).

**Anterior** muscles that dorsiflex the foot include the tibialis anterior, peroneus

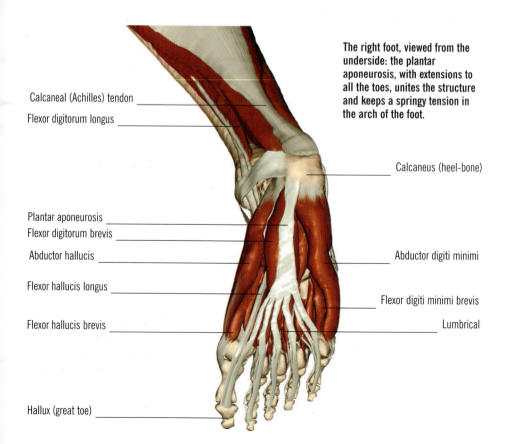

The right foot, viewed from the underside: the plantar aponeurosis, with extensions to all the toes, unites the structure and keeps a springy tension in the arch of the foot.

Calcaneal (Achilles) tendon

Flexor digitorum longus

Calcaneus (heel-bone)

Plantar aponeurosis

Flexor digitorum brevis

Abductor hallucis

Abductor digiti minimi

Flexor hallucis longus

Flexor digiti minimi brevis

Flexor hallucis brevis

Lumbrical

Hallux (great toe)

tertius, extensor digitorum longus, and
extensor hallucis longus. The tibialis
anterior is the most important in
dorsiflexion; it also supports the arch and
inverts the foot. The peroneus tertius
everts it. The extensor muscles extend the
small toes and big toe.

**The lower leg and right foot in
lateral and anterior views: the
Achilles tendon is the shared
termination of two powerful
muscles, the gastrocnemius and
soleus, which pull on the
calcaneus to raise the body up
on the toes. Binding everything
in place at the ankle are two
fibrous straps, the superior and
inferior extensor retinaculum.**

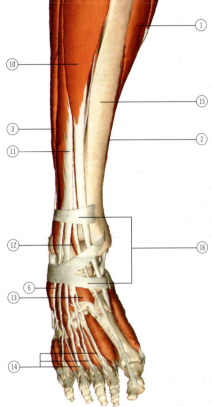

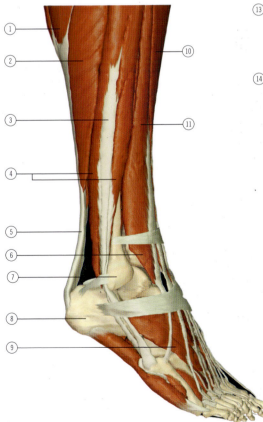

**Key**

① Gastrocnemius
② Soleus
③ Peroneus longus
④ Peroneus brevis
⑤ Calcaneal (Achilles) tendon
⑥ Personeus tertius
⑦ Fibula
⑧ Calcaneus (heel-bone)
⑨ Extensor digitorum brevis
⑩ Tibialis anterior
⑪ Extensor digitorum longus
⑫ Extensor hallucis longus
⑬ Extensor hallucis brevis
⑭ Tendons of extensor digitorum
   longus
⑮ Tibia
⑯ Extensor retinacula

# THE NERVOUS SYSTEM

THE NERVOUS SYSTEM IS THE "WIRING" of the body. It consists of trillions of interconnected nerve cells, in the brain and throughout the body, that transmit messages by means of electrical signals. It is not only responsible for thought, feeling, and activity, but also for maintaining internal balance and stability, or **homeostasis**.

The nervous system has two components. The central nervous system (CNS) consists of the brain and spinal cord. The brain is the control and processing centre of the system. An individual is consciously aware of only a small portion of the activities of the brain, which range from the maintenance and regulation of the heartbeat to the creation of a poem. Neurons in different regions of the brain deal with different kinds of information. For example, so-called vegetative (or subconscious) functions, such as the maintenance of breathing, take place in the brainstem, the part of the brain nearest the spinal cord, while the cortex, the outer part of the brain, is the site of higher-order processes. The spinal cord is the link between the brain and the body. Virtually all the body's input and output travel to the brain via the spinal cord, which is actually continuous with the brainstem.

The peripheral nervous system is defined by default: all neurons that lie outside the CNS are part of the peripheral system. It is devoted to collecting and transmitting information about the state of the body and the environment, and to sending regulatory signals to the muscles and glands. The peripheral nervous system has two divisions: the somatic nervous system and the autonomic nervous system. The somatic system supplies nerves to ("innervates") the skin, skeletal muscles, and joints, while the autonomic system supplies nerves to the body's smooth muscles, heart muscle, and viscera.

The brain, spinal cord, and peripheral nerves make up the nervous system. They form an interconnected communication network that operates by transmitting electrical signals along neural pathways.

## Key

① Cervical plexus
② Intercostal
③ Spinal cord
④ Lumbosacral plexus
⑤ Femoral
⑥ Lateral femoral cutaneous
⑦ Cerebral hemispheres
⑧ Cerebellum
⑨ Brachial plexus
⑩ Axillary
⑪ Radial
⑫ Musculocutaneous
⑬ Median
⑭ Ulnar
⑮ Sciatic
⑯ Saphenous
⑰ Common peroneal
⑱ Tibial
⑲ Superficial peroneal

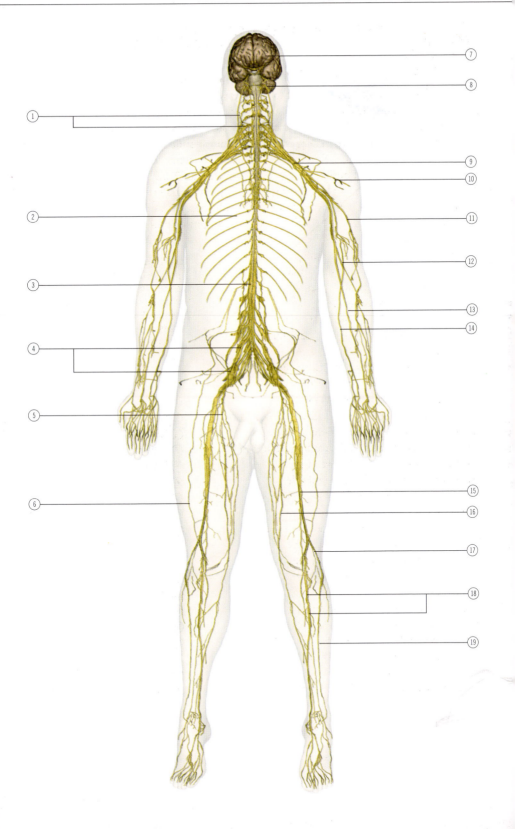

# HOW THE NERVOUS SYSTEM WORKS

BODY'S HIGH-SPEED COMMUNICATION NETWORK relies on trillions of interconnected neurons, or nerve cells. Without these it would be impossible for us to think, feel, and act.

## Neurons and neural transmission

**Neurons** are specialized cells that generate and respond to electrical signals called **nerve impulses**, or "action potentials". The **nucleus** of a neuron is contained in a cell body. Connected to the cell body are **dendrites** that carry information towards the cell body, and an **axon**, a long fibre that carries nerve impulses away from the cell body. Information is transmitted through the system by one-way communication between the axon of one neuron and the dendrite of another. When the nucleus of a neuron is sufficiently stimulated, it emits an electrical impulse that is propagated down its axon. At the end of the axon is a presynaptic vesicle or synaptic pod. When it receives a nerve impulse, the vesicle releases a chemical called a **neurotransmitter** into a small space between the sending cell and the receiving cell (the synaptic gap). Dendrites on the receiving cell detect the neurotransmitter in the gap and send signals to its cell body. If this signal excites the nucleus to its firing threshold, it emits a nerve impulse of its own that is sent along to a third neuron.

## Neural circuitry

Nerves can be classified according to function:
• neurons that connect with other nerves in the central nervous system (CNS) are

called association neurons. These comprise 90 percent of all neurons;
• sensory information from the millions of receptors throughout the body is carried in the peripheral nervous system by **sensory neurons**;
• the peripheral system also relays outputs to **effectors**, i.e., muscles and glands. The neurons that carry these outputs are called **motor neurons**.

The arrangement of neurons in the brain and spinal cord gives rise to distinct areas of gray and white matter. The gray matter is made up primarily of cell bodies and dendrites, while the white matter is composed primarily of axons and their associated structures.

Much of the peripheral nervous system is composed of bundles of nerve fibres, which are contained within protective sheaths that form tracts or cords. These are the nerves themselves. Most nerves are composed of both sensory and motor nerve fibres, carrying information both to and from the CNS.

In the nervous system, the transmission of nerve signals is mediated by synapses. The nerve signal, or action potential, arrives at the presynaptic membrane of the synaptic end-bulb. This triggers release of chemical neurotransmitters stored in membrane-bound packets called synaptic vesicles. The neurotransmitter molecules then generate a response by stimulating receptors on the postsynaptic membrane, which in the central nervous system commonly belongs to a specialized structure called a dendritic spine.

The nerves are arranged hierarchically. The large nerves emanating from the spinal cord branch into smaller ones, and these branch again until innervation (that is, nerve supply to an area) is complete.

Most neural pathways exist in pairs, with one member of the pair branching to the left-hand side of the body and the other member of the pair branching to the right-hand side. Most of these pathways cross over in the brain or spinal cord to the opposite side of the brain, with the result that sensory and motor information from one side of the body is controlled by the opposite side of the brain (something called contralateral control).

## Sensory Receptors

Detecting physical stimuli and transducing them into electrical codes that can be used by the nervous system is the task of specialized neural structures called sensory receptors. They are the first neurons in each sensory pathway. The receptors for each sense are unique, with different receptors being sensitive to different forms of energy: mechanical, thermal, chemical, or electromagnetic. The energy is transformed by the nervous system into the different sensations of vision, hearing, touch, taste, and smell. Sensory information from within the body, processed by receptors of the autonomic nervous system, usually does not give rise to conscious sensations.

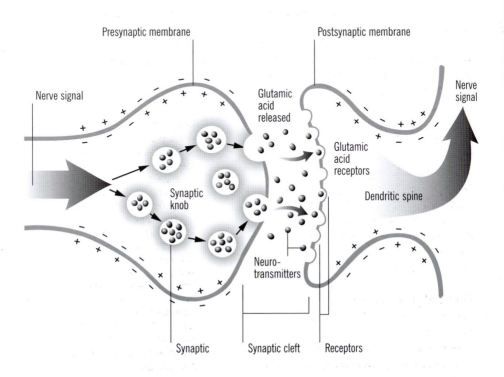

Presynaptic membrane | Postsynaptic membrane
Nerve signal | Glutamic acid released | Nerve signal
Synaptic knob | Glutamic acid receptors
Dendritic spine
Neuro-transmitters
Synaptic | Synaptic cleft | Receptors

# THE BRAIN

THE BRAIN IS THE CORE OF the nervous system; virtually all information from the senses and internal receptors flows to the brain, and all bodily activities depend on instructions from it.

The brain has three main parts: the cerebrum, the cerebellum, and the brainstem. The outer and most massive area, the cerebrum, is composed of two cerebral hemispheres, each of which is covered with a thin layer, the cerebral cortex. The corrugated surface of the cerebrum has numerous folds called **sulci** and ridges called **gyri**, enabling a larger amount of cortex to fit within the skull.

The cerebral hemispheres are divided into four lobes specialized for specific processes: the frontal, parietal, temporal, and occipital. Visual processing, for example, takes place in the occipital lobe. The cerebral hemispheres are kept in constant communication by the corpus callosum, a large bundle of nerve fibres. In the lower portion of the hemispheres is the limbic system, which is important to emotion, memory, and **homeostasis**.

The cerebellum is concerned with balance and muscular coordination. The remaining part of the brain is the brainstem. In addition to connecting the brain and spinal cord, it contains structures that regulate important internal functions such as breathing and heart rate. **Cerebrospinal fluid** surrounds the brain (and spinal cord) and fills interior brain spaces called ventricles. Its cushioning effect provides protection from injury.

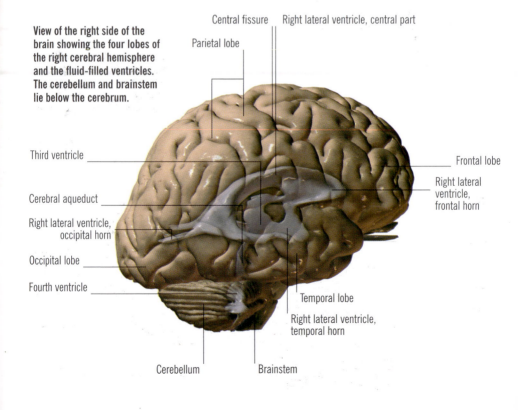

View of the right side of the brain showing the four lobes of the right cerebral hemisphere and the fluid-filled ventricles. The cerebellum and brainstem lie below the cerebrum.

Central fissure

Parietal lobe

Right lateral ventricle, central part

Third ventricle

Cerebral aqueduct

Right lateral ventricle, occipital horn

Occipital lobe

Fourth ventricle

Frontal lobe

Right lateral ventricle, frontal horn

Temporal lobe

Right lateral ventricle, temporal horn

Cerebellum

Brainstem

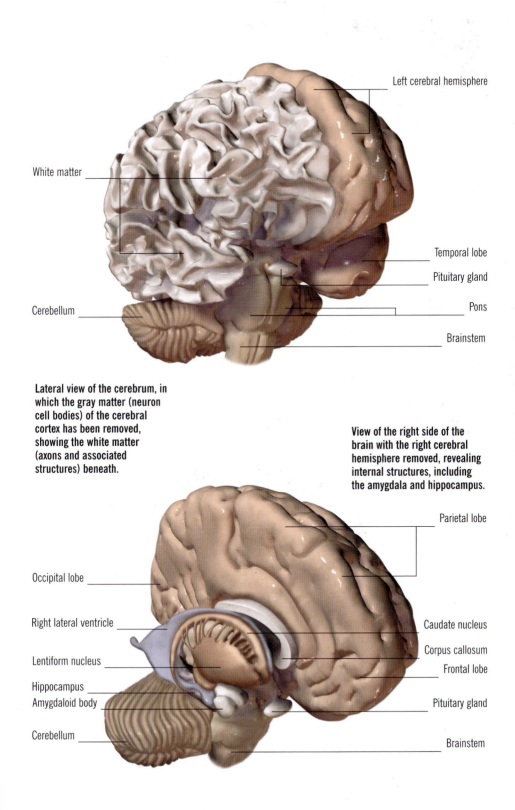

Left cerebral hemisphere

White matter

Temporal lobe

Pituitary gland

Cerebellum

Pons

Brainstem

**Lateral view of the cerebrum, in which the gray matter (neuron cell bodies) of the cerebral cortex has been removed, showing the white matter (axons and associated structures) beneath.**

**View of the right side of the brain with the right cerebral hemisphere removed, revealing internal structures, including the amygdala and hippocampus.**

Parietal lobe

Occipital lobe

Right lateral ventricle

Caudate nucleus

Corpus callosum

Lentiform nucleus

Frontal lobe

Hippocampus

Amygdaloid body

Pituitary gland

Cerebellum

Brainstem

# THE CRANIAL NERVES

THE 12 BILATERALLY SYMMETRICAL PAIRS OF cranial nerves emerge from the bottom of the brain. Some nerves contain motor and/or sensory fibres that innervate (supply nerves to) the skin and muscles of the head and neck, while others are connected with the special senses of smell, sight, hearing, balance, and taste.

The cranial nerves are labelled both by name and by number (Roman numerals are used), typically according to their primary function. Those involved with the special sense organs are the olfactory nerve (I), which projects to the nasal cavity and carries information about smell; the optic nerve (II), which travels to the eyes and relays visual information from the retinas; the vestibulocochlear nerve (VIII), which carries sensory information about both hearing and balance from the ears; and the glossopharyngeal nerve (IX), which projects to the tongue and transmits taste information, as well as controlling swallowing action.

Three of the remaining cranial nerves are involved in eye movement: the oculomotor nerve (III), the trochlear nerve (IV), and the abducens nerve (VI). The trigeminal nerve (V) relays sensory input from the eye, face, and teeth, and also controls chewing. The facial nerve (VII) controls muscles involved in facial expression. The vagus nerve (X) projects to the throat and abdomen and has a role in many involuntary functions such as the heart rate.

The accessory nerve (XI) controls large movements of the head and shoulders and also participates in vocal production. Finally, the hypoglossal nerve (XII) controls muscles in the tongue.

## The blood-brain barrier

Although the brain makes up only a small proportion of the body's total mass, it has high-energy needs and therefore receives 20 percent of the body's total blood flow. In addition to nutrients, however, the blood carries many chemicals and other substances that could interfere with electrochemical communication within the brain. Fortunately, specialized capillary walls create a blood-brain barrier that impedes the movement of most substances from the blood to the brain, while allowing small molecules such as glucose and oxygen to pass through freely. Despite its usefulness, the blood-brain barrier prevents some potentially beneficial drugs, such as antibiotics, from entering the brain, and permits the passage of some potentially harmful substances, such as alcohol.

**A view of the underside of the brain showing the attachment points of the cranial nerves.**

**Key**
1. Optic nerve (II)
2. Optic chiasma
3. Trochlear nerve (IV)
4. Cerebellum
5. Right cerebral hemisphere
6. Olfactory nerve (I)
7. Oculomotor nerve (III)
8. Trigeminal nerve (V)
9. Abducens nerve (VI)
10. Facial (VII), Vestibulocochlear (VIII), Glossopharyngeal (IX), and Vagus (X) nerves
11. Hypoglossal nerve (XII)
12. Accessory nerve (XI)
13. Medulla oblongata

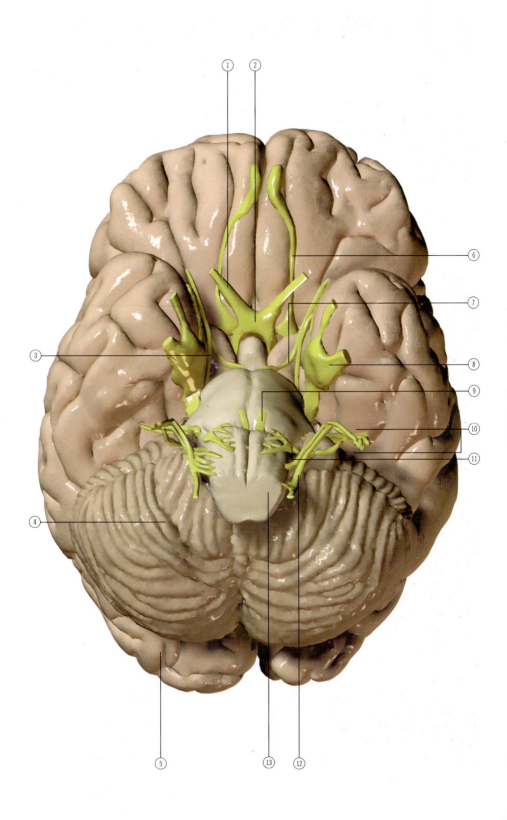

# THE SPINAL CORD

THE SPINAL CORD RELAYS INFORMATION BETWEEN the brain and body. Continuous with the brainstem, it extends through the foramen magnum, down through a protective channel formed by the vertebrae of the backbone to the first lumbar vertebra. The cord is divided crosswise into 31 segments, each of which gives rise to a pair of bilaterally symmetrical spinal nerves. These emerge from the cord through gaps between the vertebrae. The spinal nerves pass sensory and motor information from the spinal cord to a particular segment of the body.

Within the spinal cord, the gray matter forms an H-shaped central core. The white matter forms long pathways called tracts. Ascending tracts are formed by sensory nerve fibres (**axons**) and carry sensory information to the brain. Descending tracts of motor nerve fibres convey motor output from the brain.

The spinal nerves branch off at various points to form other peripheral nerves, which branch in turn to complete the system of wiring that innervates the body.

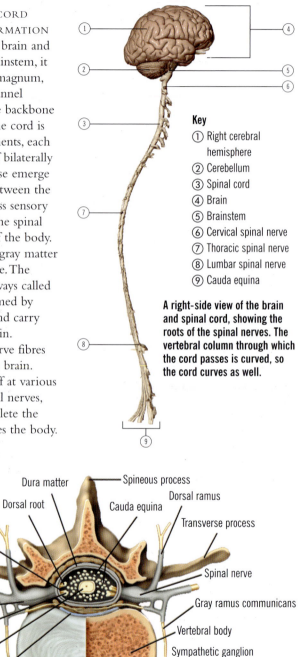

**Key**
1. Right cerebral hemisphere
2. Cerebellum
3. Spinal cord
4. Brain
5. Brainstem
6. Cervical spinal nerve
7. Thoracic spinal nerve
8. Lumbar spinal nerve
9. Cauda equina

A right-side view of the brain and spinal cord, showing the roots of the spinal nerves. The vertebral column through which the cord passes is curved, so the cord curves as well.

A cross-section showing the relationship of the vertebrae and the spinal cord.

Dura matter
Spineous process
Dorsal root
Dorsal ramus
Cauda equina
Arachnoid
Transverse process
Ventral ramus
Spinal nerve
Spinal ganglion
Gray ramus communicans
Ventral root
Vertebral body
Spinal cord
Sympathetic ganglion
Posterior longitudinal ligament
Anterior longitudinal ligament
Interventral disc

# THE AUTONOMIC NERVOUS SYSTEM

THE AUTONOMIC NERVOUS SYSTEM (ANS) controls smooth muscles, heart muscle, and the glands. It automatically and continuously regulates the internal environment of the body to a steady state (**homeostasis**) as internal or external conditions change.

The ANS is a motor system, though unlike the somatic nervous system, which is largely voluntary, the ANS is largely involuntary. Also, while the somatic motor neurons project directly from the central nervous system (CNS) to the muscles they control, in the ANS, a **preganglionic** neuron projects from the CNS to a **ganglion** (swelling), where it synapses with a second neuron (**postganglionic** neuron) that projects to the target effector. The sympathetic and parasympathetic divisions of the ANS (see box) follow separate pathways through the body. Sympathetic system neurons leave the CNS from segments in the middle of the spinal cord, while those of the parasympathetic system emerge from the brainstem and lower spinal cord. The ganglia on which the preganglionic neurons of the sympathetic system synapse form a chain adjacent to the spinal cord, whereas the parasympathetic ganglia are within or near their effectors.

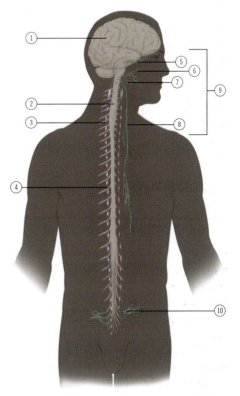

Diagram of ANS connections with the brain and spinal cord, showing nerves of the sympathetic division.

**Key**
1. Brain
2. Spinal cord
3. Paravertebral (chain) ganglion
4. Sympathetic trunk or chain
5. Oculomotor nerves (III)
6. Facial nerves (VII)
7. Glossopharyngeal nerves (IX)
8. Vagus nerves
9. Cranial parasympathetic outflow
10. Pelvic splanchnic nerves (sacral parasympathetic outflow)

## The sympathetic and parasympathetic systems

The divisions of the ANS, the sympathetic and parasympathetic nervous systems, have complementary functions. The sympathetic nervous system prepares the body to cope with sudden changes, usually by stimulating effectors, as when the heart rate increases in preparation for stress. The parasympathetic system regulates most involuntary functions under normal conditions, and usually decreases the activity of effectors.

# THE MAJOR NERVE BUNDLES

A NERVE PLEXUS IS A BUNDLE, or network, of nerves that originates in a particular region of the body. The largest plexi are the brachial and lumbosacral. Both consist of branches of several spinal nerves that converge in the plexus and give rise to the nerves that supply the extremities.

## The brachial and lumbosacral nerves

The brachial plexus is formed by nerves that innervate (supply nerves to) the chest and arms; the lumbosacral plexus is composed of two separate plexi, the lumbar and sacral plexi. The nerves of the lumbar plexus serve the thigh, while the sacral plexus comprises nerves to the buttocks, leg, and foot. There are numerous other plexi in the body; for example, the cardiac plexus, which is a network of autonomic nerve fibres at the base of the heart.

Formed from branches of the fifth to eighth cervical and first thoracic nerves, the brachial plexus is located in the posterior triangle of the neck, between the clavicle and the sternocleidomastoid muscle. It divides into two main sets of

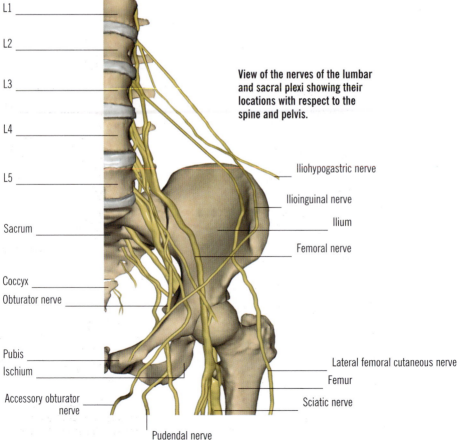

L1

L2

L3

L4

L5

Sacrum

Coccyx

Obturator nerve

Pubis

Ischium

Accessory obturator nerve

**View of the nerves of the lumbar and sacral plexi showing their locations with respect to the spine and pelvis.**

Iliohypogastric nerve

Ilioinguinal nerve

Ilium

Femoral nerve

Lateral femoral cutaneous nerve

Femur

Sciatic nerve

Pudendal nerve

branches: the supraclavicular, which innervates parts of the chest and the upper back; and the infraclavicular, which innervates the remaining parts of the chest and the arms. When the arm is at rest, the cords of the brachial plexus can be detected beneath the skin by running a hand along the curvature of the second rib.

The lumbar plexus, created from branches of the first three lumbar nerves, is situated on the posterior abdominal wall among the fibres of the psoas major muscle. From it arise the femoral nerve, serving the muscles and skin of the anterior thigh; the obturator nerve,

innervating the adductor muscles and the skin of the medial thigh; and the lateral femoral cutaneous nerves, serving the skin of the lateral thigh.

The sacral plexus—with branches of the fourth and fifth lumbar nerves and the first three sacral nerves—lies below the lumbar plexus, against the **posterior** and **lateral** portions of the pelvis. This bundle gives rise to the sciatic nerve, which innervates the leg and foot. Also emanating from the sacral plexus are the nerves that supply the hamstrings, the gluteal muscles, and the skin of the buttocks and part of the thigh.

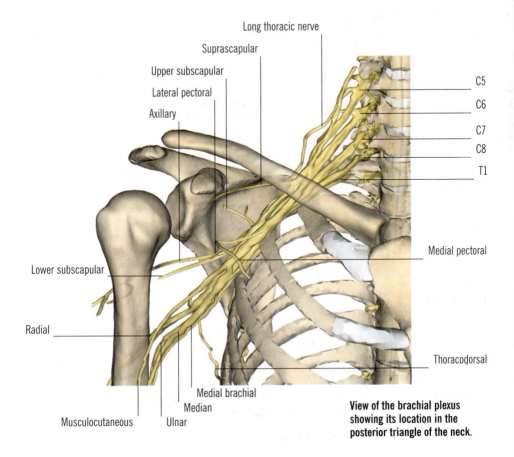

Long thoracic nerve
Suprascapular
Upper subscapular
Lateral pectoral
Axillary
C5
C6
C7
C8
T1
Lower subscapular
Medial pectoral
Radial
Thoracodorsal
Medial brachial
Median
Musculocutaneous
Ulnar

**View of the brachial plexus showing its location in the posterior triangle of the neck.**

# THE EYE

THE EYE IS A HOLLOW SPHERE that detects light. Light enters through the cornea, passes through the focusing lens, and is projected onto the back of the eye, where it is detected by light–sensitive cells and converted into nerve impulses. Signals are then sent through the optic nerve to the brain, where they undergo further processing in specialized visual areas before conscious "seeing" occurs.

Each eye lies on a cushion of fat within the orbit, or socket, of the skull. The eyeball is moved by six extrinsic muscles that run from the orbit to the sclera, the white of the eye. Four rectus muscles move the eyeball straight up and down, and from side to side; the two oblique muscles move the eye up and down at an angle. The lacrimal glands, set within the orbit above the eyeball, continuously secrete dilute saline tears.

The sclera forms most of the outer layer of the eyeball. At the front is a clear

**Key**

① Superior rectus muscle
② Lateral rectus muscle
③ Optic nerve
④ Inferior rectus muscle
⑤ Eyeball
⑥ Cornea
⑦ Sclera
⑧ Inferior oblique muscle
⑨ Skull

**A diagram of the eyeball (below) showing its three layers, and the jellylike vitreous body between the lens and retina. The optic nerve exits the eye at the optic disk, near the centre of the retina. There are no photo-receptors on the retina at the optic disk; the result is a blind spot in the visual field. There is normally no awareness of this blank spot in visual space because the brain fills it in.**

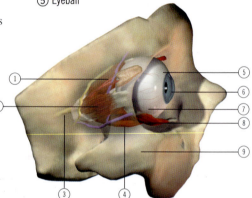

**View of the eyeball (above) situated within the orbit of the skull. Just a sixth of the eyeball can actually be seen.**

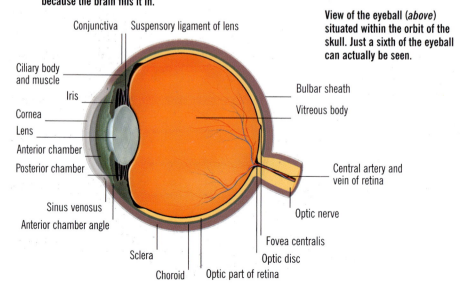

Conjunctiva
Suspensory ligament of lens
Ciliary body and muscle
Iris
Cornea
Lens
Anterior chamber
Posterior chamber
Sinus venosus
Anterior chamber angle
Sclera
Choroid
Optic part of retina
Optic disc
Fovea centralis
Optic nerve
Central artery and vein of retina
Vitreous body
Bulbar sheath

region in the sclera, the cornea. A thin membrane, the conjunctiva, covers the front surface of the eye and the back of the eyelid. The coloured ring of the iris widens or narrows sphincterlike—it has two very fine muscles—making a variable aperture, the pupil, in front of the eye's lens; this regulates the amount of light entering the eye. The lens, lying behind the iris, is suspended and held in place by ligaments and the associated ciliary muscle, which alters the shape of the lens. The inner layer of the eye is the retina.

Nerve impulses from the eyes travel to the visual cortex, where conscious "seeing" occurs. After they pass into the brain, some of the nerve fibres from each eye cross over and join with the noncrossing nerve fibres from the other eye to form two optic tracts, each with information from both eyes. One tract goes to the right primary visual area, the other to the left. The primary visual areas are located in the occipital lobes at the back of the left and right cerebral hemispheres. Here, different regions are specialized for processing different kinds of visual information, such as shape, size, colour, and motion.

## Rods and cones

The optic retina covers the back of the eye. It contains two types of photoreceptors: **rods** and **cones**. Cones are concentrated in a small central area behind the lens, the **macula lutea**; the rest of the retina contains only rods. Rods are specialized for night vision, and, because of their location, provide **peripheral vision**. They give rise only to **monochrome** images. Cones, specialized for day vision, detect colour and provide more visual detail.

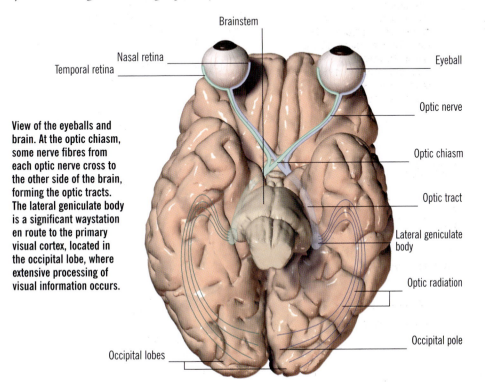

**View of the eyeballs and brain. At the optic chiasm, some nerve fibres from each optic nerve cross to the other side of the brain, forming the optic tracts. The lateral geniculate body is a significant waystation en route to the primary visual cortex, located in the occipital lobe, where extensive processing of visual information occurs.**

Brainstem

Nasal retina

Temporal retina

Eyeball

Optic nerve

Optic chiasm

Optic tract

Lateral geniculate body

Optic radiation

Occipital pole

Occipital lobes

# THE EAR

THE EAR IS THE SENSE ORGAN that detects soundwaves in the air and transforms them into nerve impulses which are ultimately interpreted by the brain as sound. The ears also contain structures that sense the position of the body, head, and eyes relative to the external world, and are critical for maintaining balance.

Incoming soundwaves travelling through the air are directed into the auditory canal by the pinna of the outer ear. The tympanic membrane, or eardrum, stretched over the end of the canal, vibrates in response to the soundwaves. This vibration is transmitted to the three tiny bones called ossicles located in the middle ear cavity. The innermost ossicle, the stirrup (stapes) is attached to the oval window, the boundary between the middle ear and the fluid-filled inner ear. As it vibrates it pushes in and out on the window, which carries vibrations through the fluid in the inner ear.

The cochlea, the snail-shaped part of the inner ear, contains the **organ of Corti**, where the auditory receptor cells, the hair cells, are located. When a hair cell is stimulated by vibration, nerve impulses are sent through the cochlear division of the vestibulocochlear nerve to the thalamus. From there, the information travels to the primary association area of

**Front view of the ear showing parts of the pinna—the only visible portion of the ear. The ear canal funnels soundwaves to the eardrum, the ossicles, and the inner ear.**

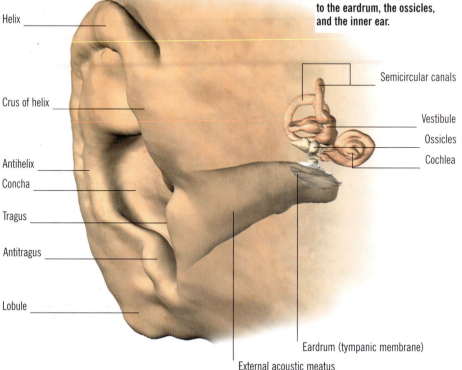

Helix

Crus of helix

Antihelix

Concha

Tragus

Antitragus

Lobule

Semicircular canals

Vestibule

Ossicles

Cochlea

Eardrum (tympanic membrane)

External acoustic meatus
(ear canal)

the auditory cortex, located at the upper edge of the temporal lobes, where it is consciously perceived.

Some nerve fibres from each ear cross over and pass to the primary auditory area of the cerebral hemisphere on the opposite side, so that each area receives inputs from each ear. Separate regions in the auditory cortex process separate characteristics of auditory inputs, such as pitch and loudness. The adjacent auditory association area classifies the sound as speech, music, or simply as noise.

## Key
① Semicircular canals
② Lateral semicircular canal
③ Incus
④ Malleus
⑤ Tympanic membrane
⑥ Stapes
⑦ Anterior semicircular canal
⑧ Posterior semicircular canal
⑨ Vestibule
⑩ Vestibulocochlear nerve
⑪ Cochlea

## Balance

The ear helps the body maintain its spatial equilibrium. The inner ear contains three fluid-filled semicircular canals, set at approximately right angles to each other. At the base of each is an **ampulla**, within which are sensory hairs embedded in a gelatinous substance called the **cupula**. When the head moves, fluid pressure in the semicircular canals changes minutely and the cupula is deformed somewhat; the embedded hair cells respond to these movements. Combined inputs from the ampullae allow detection of movement in any direction.

The central portion of the inner ear, the **vestibule**, contains two other balance detectors, the **utricle** and **saccule**, which also use hair cells—in a slightly different way from ampullae—to detect changes in the orientation of the head. Balance-related information is transmitted via nerve impulses originating in the hair cells through the vestibular division of the vestibulocochlear nerve to various areas of the central nervous system (CNS).

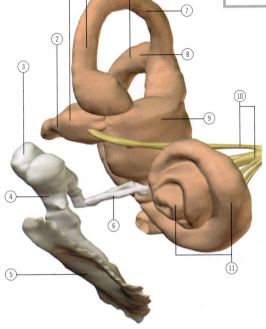

A view of the ossicles and the inner ear with skin and muscles removed. Soundwaves pass along the ossicles, which send vibrations through the oval window into the inner ear. Here they are converted into electrical signals and passed to the brain along the vestibulocochlear nerve. The semicircular canals and other structures in the vestibule sense changes in position and help the body maintain equilibrium.

# THE NOSE

IN BREATHING, AS AIR PASSES THROUGH the nose, it is filtered, warmed, and humidified. The incoming air also carries chemicals that are detected by sensory receptors high in the walls of the nasal passages. These olfactory (smell) receptors can register thousands of different smells and are sensitive enough to detect molecules the concentration of which is just a few parts per trillion.

The external nose consists of the nasal bone, attached to the frontal bone, and flexible cartilage below. The nostrils, or external nares, are the openings located on either side of the nasal septum, a structure composed of cartilage that bisects vertically both the external nose and the nasal cavity. The nasal cavity is behind, and open to, the external nose. It is bounded by the ethmoid and sphenoid bones at the top and the palate below. At the back, the nasal cavity opens into the upper pharynx (throat) through the internal nares.

The millions of **olfactory** chemoreceptors are located only in the olfactory epithelium, a yellowish patch of about one square inch (6 sq cm) on the roof and adjoining walls of each side of the nasal cavity. These receptors detect airborne chemicals dissolved in the

**Side view of the head, with concha exposed, clearly detailing the olfactory nerve, the first of the cranial nerves.**

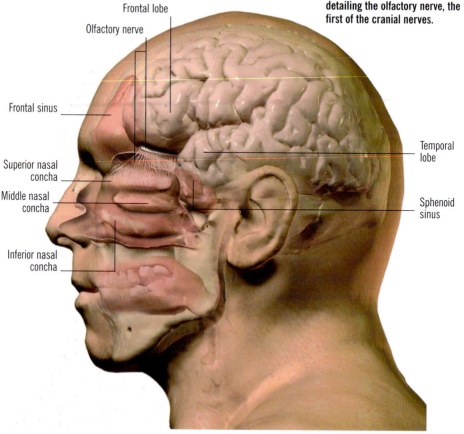

Frontal lobe

Olfactory nerve

Frontal sinus

Superior nasal concha

Middle nasal concha

Inferior nasal concha

Temporal lobe

Sphenoid sinus

watery mucous secreted by membranes within the nasal cavity.

Nerve impulses from the olfactory chemoreceptors travel directly to the cortex. Their **axons** collect into small bundles, forming the olfactory nerve that passes through holes in the cribriform ("sievelike") plate of the ethmoid bone. The individual nerve fibres synapse on the olfactory bulb, which is located on the underside of the frontal lobe.

Nerve tracts **originating** at the olfactory bulb pass both to the olfactory cortex and to the nearby amygdala, a structure that is known to be involved in emotion and memory. This latter pathway may be responsible for the poignant memories that familiar smells sometimes trigger.

**Key**
1. Superior concha
2. Middle concha
3. Inferior concha
4. Superior meatus
5. Middle meatus
6. Inferior meatus
7. Frontal paranasal sinus
8. Nasal cavity
9. Left external nares
10. Opening of auditory (eustachian tube)
11. Nasopharynx

**Side view of the nose showing the nasal cavity and the nasal epithelium, the sensory area where smell is detected.**

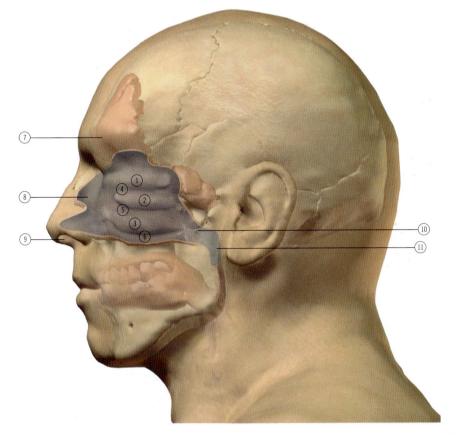

# THE ENDOCRINE SYSTEM

THE ENDOCRINE SYSTEM IS A CHEMICAL communication system that controls a variety of activities in the body at the cellular level. It is made up of glands in the head and trunk that secrete gland-specific **hormones**. These help to coordinate and control functions including growth, sexual development, and response to danger.

The endocrine system shares certain properties with the nervous system, the body's other internal communication mechanism. Both transmit signals to distant sites and get feedback from their targets, but they function very differently. The nervous system uses electrical signals to send messages along nerve fibres to specific destinations; the endocrine system sends hormonal messages to all parts of the body through the bloodstream. However, hormones affect areas only where there are hormone-specific receptor cells to which they can attach.

The binding of hormone to receptor triggers reactions within a cell that affect its function. Some hormones influence many cells, others act in limited areas. Unlike electrical impulses of the nervous system, the effects of which can occur almost instantaneously and are typically of short duration, hormones take time to work and can have long-term effects.

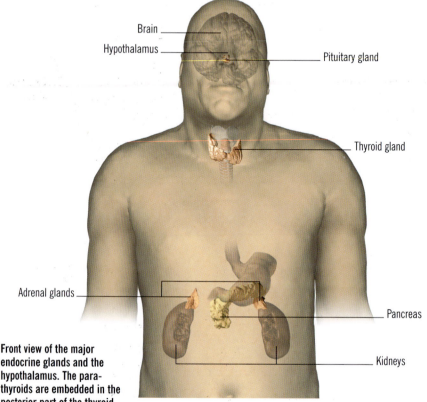

Brain

Hypothalamus

Pituitary gland

Thyroid gland

Adrenal glands

Pancreas

Kidneys

**Front view of the major endocrine glands and the hypothalamus. The para-thyroids are embedded in the posterior part of the thyroid.**

Hormone-mediated activities are quite sensitive to the blood level of a specific hormone to which they react. If too much or too little hormone is present, disruption of normal processes occurs. The main mechanism for maintaining the proper level of a hormone is a negative feedback loop in which changes in blood levels of a hormone signal to an endocrine gland or other organ to increase or decrease its activity. These loops can involve more than one hormone and more than one gland. For example, regulation of thyroid secretions involves the hypothalamus as well as the pituitary gland.

## The endocrine glands

There are two kinds of glands in the body, both of which release secretions. **Exocrine** glands secrete substances, for example, saliva and sweat, through ducts opening to a bodily surface. Conversely, glands in the **endocrine** system do not use ducts, but secrete hormones straight into the bloodstream. The major endocrine glands are the pituitary, pineal, thyroid, parathyroids, and adrenal. Areas of the pancreas, ovaries, and testes also act as endocrine glands. In addition, the hypothalamus, a region of the brain, secretes hormones that regulate the operation of the pituitary gland.

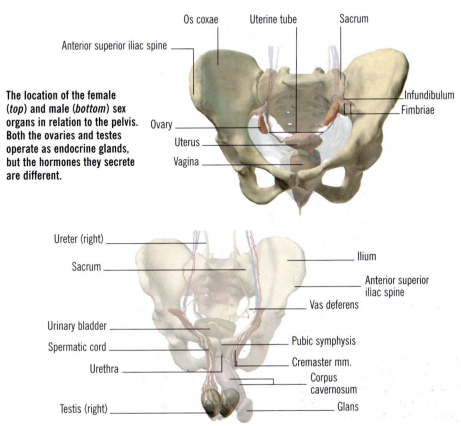

**The location of the female (*top*) and male (*bottom*) sex organs in relation to the pelvis. Both the ovaries and testes operate as endocrine glands, but the hormones they secrete are different.**

Os coxae
Uterine tube
Sacrum
Anterior superior iliac spine
Infundibulum
Fimbriae
Ovary
Uterus
Vagina

Ureter (right)
Sacrum
Ilium
Anterior superior iliac spine
Vas deferens
Urinary bladder
Spermatic cord
Urethra
Pubic symphysis
Cremaster mm.
Corpus cavernosum
Testis (right)
Glans

# THE HYPOTHALAMUS AND PITUITARY

THE HYPOTHALAMUS IS THE REGION OF the brain—located in the middle at its base—that controls bodily functions related to **homeostasis**, or internal stability. In addition to its role in the endocrine system, the hypothalamus regulates many functions of the autonomic nervous system (ANS).

A pea-sized organ, the pituitary gland lies immediately beneath the hypothalamus, in a depression of the base of the skull, and is connected to the hypothalamus by a stalk. The pituitary gland releases a number of hormones that in many cases affect other endocrine glands—and release of these pituitary hormones is controlled, in turn, by the hypothalamus.

The pituitary gland has two functionally distinct lobes, the anterior and posterior, which secrete different hormones and interact with the hypothalamus in different ways.

## Anterior lobe hormones

Secretions of the anterior lobe are controlled by hormones sent from the hypothalamus, called releasing hormones and inhibiting hormones. They are carried directly to the anterior pituitary lobe by means of hypothalamic-hypophyseal portal veins. Specific hypothalamic hormones bind to receptors on specific anterior pituitary cells, modulating the release of the hormone they produce.

The major anterior lobe hormones, their target sites, and the effects they stimulate are:

- thyroid-stimulating hormone (TSH)—thyroid gland: release of thyroid hormone;
- adrenocorticotropic hormone (ACTH)—adrenal glands: release of glucocorticoid hormones;
- growth hormone—body: growth in children and adolescents;
- follicle-stimulating hormone (FSH)—ovaries: egg maturation and release of oestrogen; testes: sperm production;
- luteinizing hormone (LH)—ovaries: ovulation and progesterone production; testes: testosterone production;
- prolactin—mammary glands: milk production.

## Posterior lobe hormones

Hormones released by the posterior lobe originate in the hypothalamus itself. The posterior lobe is largely made up of the axons of hypothalamic neurons. These have special nerve fibres that are used to transport hormones to the posterior lobe, where they will be stored until a nerve impulse stimulates their release.

The posterior lobe hormones, their target sites, and their effects are:

- oxytocin—uterus: stimulates contractions in childbirth; mammary glands: release of milk;
- prolactin—mammary glands: milk production;
- antidiuretic hormones (ADH)—kidneys: reduces volume of urine.

## Hormone level controls

Hormone levels are mostly maintained by negative feedback, which lowers hormone secretion if the physiological response becomes excessive. This type of control uses hormones, the nervous system, or chemical stimuli to send feedback signals to the hormone-releasing tissues.

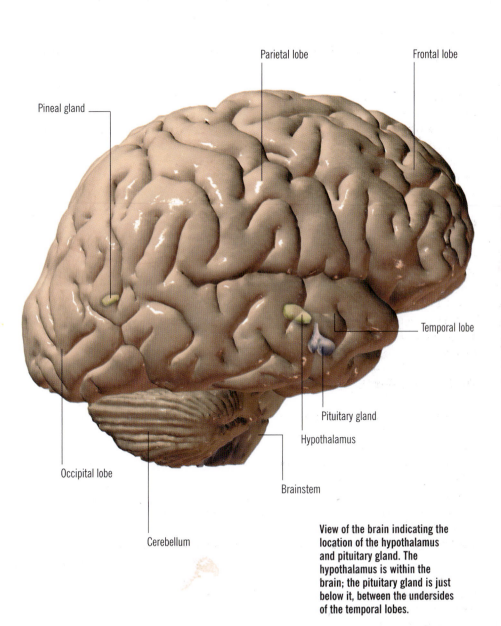

Parietal lobe

Frontal lobe

Pineal gland

Temporal lobe

Pituitary gland

Hypothalamus

Occipital lobe

Brainstem

Cerebellum

View of the brain indicating the location of the hypothalamus and pituitary gland. The hypothalamus is within the brain; the pituitary gland is just below it, between the undersides of the temporal lobes.

# THE THYROID AND PARATHYROIDS

THE THYROID GLAND, LOCATED BELOW THE voice box, is the largest organ with purely endocrine functions. It secretes thyroid hormone, which accelerates the speed of energy-consuming reactions inside the body (that is, it raises the metabolic rate). The thyroid and the four pea-sized parathyroids embedded in its surface also secrete hormones that regulate calcium levels.

**Thyroid hormone** is the collective name for two hormones: **thyroxine** (T4) and **triiodothyronine** (T3)—the latter is more active than T4 but is present in much smaller quantities. The hormone's makeup requires iodine, obtained from food and water; it is the body's only use of that element. In addition to increasing metabolic activity in cells, thyroid hormone is important for growth, and is necessary for the normal operation of the heart and nervous system.

The thyroid also secretes a third hormone, **calcitonin**. Together with **parathyroid hormone** (PTH) secreted by the parathyroids, calcitonin regulates the level of calcium circulating in the blood. Calcium is used in nerve impulse transmission and blood clotting, as well as muscle contraction.

When there is too much calcium, the excess is used to create bone. Conversely, when the calcium level is too low, calcium in bones is broken down, or reabsorbed, and returned to the bloodstream. Calcitonin is the hormone that lowers the blood level of calcium by promoting its uptake into bone and slowing its withdrawal back to the blood. Parathyroid hormone has the opposite effect, acting when more calcium is needed in the bloodstream, for example, by stimulating the uptake of calcium from food during digestion.

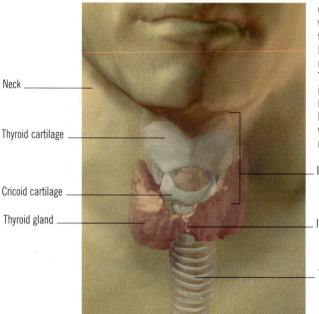

Neck

Thyroid cartilage

Cricoid cartilage

Thyroid gland

Curving around the front of the trachea slightly below the larynx, the thyroid resembles a butterfly, having two lobes connected by a much smaller central section. The parathyroid glands are set into the back part of the thyroid. If sufficient dietary iodine is lacking, the thyroid enlarges, which causes a swelling in the neck called a goitre.

Larynx

Isthmus

Trachea

# THE ADRENALS

THE ADRENAL GLANDS ARE SITUATED ON top of the kidneys, encased in a connective tissue capsule and cushioned in a layer of fat. Each consists of an outer section, the cortex, and an inner section, the medulla. The cortex releases several **corticosteroid** hormones, while the medulla produces **epinephrine** (**adrenaline**) and **norepinephrine** (**noradrenaline**).

The adrenal cortex produces three distinct classes of hormones. The first, **glucocorticoids**, regulate glucose levels and affect cellular processes. The major glucocorticoid in human beings is **cortisol**. Its release is controlled by **adrenocorticotropic hormone** (ACTH), which originates from the pituitary gland. Cortisol increases glucose levels, and also helps the body cope with causes of stress such as trauma, bleeding, and infection.

The second, **mineralocorticoids**, control the levels of potassium and sodium circulating in the body. For example, the hormone **aldosterone** prevents sodium excretion by the kidneys. Stable concentrations of potassium and sodium are vital for transmitting nerve impulses, regulating blood pressure and volume, and for muscle contraction.

The third type, the primary **gonadocorticoids**, are masculinizing hormones, or **androgens**. Adrenal androgens have minimal effects on males, since androgens are released in much larger amounts by the testes. In women, they promote sexual behaviour and cause the growth of pubic and underarm hair.

The hormones of the medulla, epinephrine and norepinephrine, are responsible for the "fight or flight" reaction to sudden stress. When released, they prepare the body to fight or flee by directing blood towards the skeletal muscles, speeding up the heart and breathing rates, and increasing the amount of available glucose. When stimulation by the autonomic nervous system ceases, release of the hormones stops, and their effects subside.

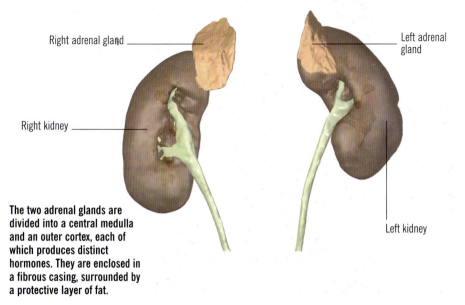

Right adrenal gland

Right kidney

Left adrenal gland

Left kidney

The two adrenal glands are divided into a central medulla and an outer cortex, each of which produces distinct hormones. They are enclosed in a fibrous casing, surrounded by a protective layer of fat.

# THE PANCREAS

THE PANCREAS IS LOCATED ACROSS THE back of the abdomen, lying behind and partially concealed by the stomach, at the level of the 1st and 2nd lumbar vertebrae. It consists of a head, neck, and tail, its head being tucked into the curve formed by the duodenum, the initial part of the small intestine. Its tail rests against the spleen. The pancreas plays a role in both the digestion process and hormone production.

## Dual function

Most of the pancreas functions as an **exocrine** gland, secreting digestive enzymes in the pancreatic juice through ducts into the adjacent duodenum. The alkaline pancreatic juice contains four enzymes: trypsin, chymotrypsin, amylase, and lipase.

However, the pancreas also releases two **endocrine** hormones that regulate blood sugar (glucose) levels. A stable, steady supply of glucose must be available to provide the energy that cells need to function properly. When levels are too high or too low, uptake of glucose by the cells is impaired. Large fluctuations in blood glucose levels can cause convulsions and even coma.

Some glucose is stored in the body in the form of **glycogen**, a complex carbohydrate composed of glucose molecules. If blood glucose levels become too low, alpha cells in the pancreatic islets (*see box*) secrete more glucagon hormone, which stimulates the liver to break down glycogen into glucose. The glucose passes into the bloodstream, restoring the body's proper balance.

Conversely, if the level of blood glucose becomes high, as is the case after meals, beta cells in the pancreatic islets secrete insulin. Insulin decreases the level of glucose in the blood by stimulating its uptake or use by the skeletal muscles, liver, and **adipose** (fat) cells. Glucose taken up by the skeletal muscles is either expended in movement or converted to glycogen and stored. Glucose travelling to the liver is converted to glycogen. The glucose taken up by adipose cells is either used in cell metabolism or stored as fat. When sufficient glucose has been removed from the blood, insulin secretion by the pancreatic islet drops off.

## Islets of Langerhans

The majority of the pancreatic volume (99 percent) is occupied by glandular tissue that secretes pancreatic juice containing digestive enzymes. Since the pancreatic juice passes via a series of pancreatic ducts into the intestinal tube, this glandular tissue is classified as exocrine. The pancreas also produces the hormones insulin and glucagon, which are produced from tiny clusters of cells called islets of Langerhans. As this hormonal release occurs directly into the bloodstream, the islets are classified as endocrine. There are about one million islets spread throughout the exocrine tissue, but remarkably they form only one percent of the total pancreatic volume.

Insulin and glucagon affect glucose use and storage, and ensure that the body has sufficient fuel to supply its cells with enough energy to fuction normally. During starvation, glucagon mobilizes glucose stores, mainining the level of bloody glucose needed for brain functioning. Crucially, if insulin-secreting cells are destroyed, early-onset (type I) diabetes develops.

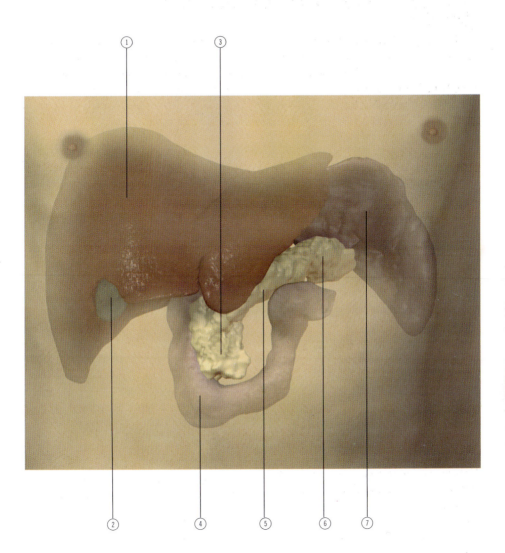

The large head of the pancreas is situated within the loop formed by the duodenum; its body and narrow tail extend across the underside of the stomach and part of the spleen.

**Key**
1. Liver
2. Gallbladder
3. Head of pancreas
4. Duodenum
5. Body of pancreas
6. Tail of pancreas
7. Spleen

# THE OVARIES

THE TWO OVARIES ARE LOCATED IN the pelvic cavity on either side of the uterus. They are held in place by pelvic and uterine ligaments. In addition to being repositories and incubators of **oocytes** (eggs), the ovaries function as endocrine glands, secreting the female sex hormones oestrogen and progesterone. A rise in oestrogen levels at **puberty** stimulates the development of characteristically female breasts and hips as well as the start of the monthly reproductive cycle. Hormone release by the ovaries declines after the menopause.

During the fertile years, oestrogen and progesterone, along with the anterior pituitary hormones follicle-stimulating hormone (FSH) and luteinizing hormone (LH), regulate the monthly reproductive cycle. The two pituitary hormones in turn stimulate the release of oestrogen and progesterone by the ovaries.

At the beginning of the ovarian cycle (the part of the reproductive cycle in which an ovum is released), FSH stimulates the release of oestrogen, which promotes the growth of oocytes in the follicles of the ovary. Oestrogen production increases further shortly before ovulation. This increase is detected by the hypothalamus, which releases more gonadotropins, causing an LH surge from the pituitary. This surge causes the mature oocyte to enlarge and be released from the ovary. As oestrogen and progesterone levels continue to rise, they inhibit both the secretion of gonadotropin-releasing hormone by the hypothalamus and of LH and FSH by the pituitary.

If no pregnancy occurs, concentrations of oestrogen and progesterone fall, stopping the inhibition, so that levels of FSH and LH can rise again to initiate the next cycle.

View of the pelvic cavity showing the ovaries and other female sex organs. Oestrogen and progesterone secreted by the ovaries trigger sexual maturity and maintain fertility until the menopause.

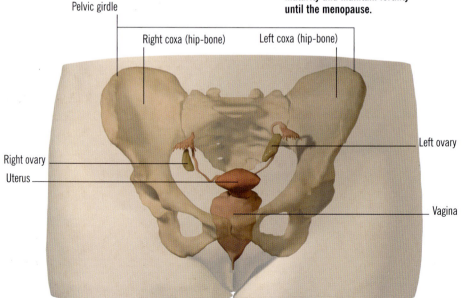

Pelvic girdle

Right coxa (hip-bone)    Left coxa (hip-bone)

Left ovary

Right ovary

Uterus

Vagina

# THE TESTES

THE TESTES, THE MAJOR MALE SEX organs, are paired, rounded structures located in the scrotum. Each testicle is covered by a sac beneath which each testis is surrounded by a thick capsule of connective tissue. As well as producing sperm, the testes release male sex hormones (androgens), most importantly testosterone, which is needed for sperm production. Sperm is made in the seminiferous tubules. Surrounding these tubules are the endocrine cells that release androgens into the bloodstream.

The testes are present in the body at birth but do not produce sperm until adolescence. When puberty sets in, testosterone production increases and stimulates the growth and maturation of the reproductive system. Maturity is reached as functional sperm is produced.

The endocrine cells within the testes are called **interstitial**, or **Leydig** cells. They produce over 95 percent of testosterone in a man.

Endocrine hormones control the male reproductive system, as they do the female system, but the male process is simpler. The hypothalamus secretes gonadotropin-releasing hormone (GnRH) from puberty. GnRH circulates to the anterior pituitary, where it causes luteinizing hormone (LH) to be released into the bloodstream. LH stimulates the interstitial cells to produce and secrete testosterone, which promotes sperm creation in the seminiferous tubules. An elevated testosterone level provides negative feedback to the anterior pituitary and hypothalamus causing decreases in GnRH and LH release; low levels have the opposite effect. Thus, a fertile level of sperm is maintained at all times. Another anterior pituitary hormone, FSH (follicle-stimulating hormone), also promotes sperm production.

**The testes hang outside and below the pelvic cavity, within the scrotum. The spermatic cord contains the blood vessels into which hormones in the testes are released and carried away from the testes.**

Right coxa (hip-bone)

Urinary bladder

Spermatic cord

Right testis

Left coxa (hip-bone)

Penis

Left testis

# THE CARDIOVASCULAR SYSTEM

MAKING UP THE BODY'S CIRCULATORY SYSTEM are three main components: a network of tubing (the veins and arteries), a pump (the heart), and circulating fluid (the blood). The veins and arteries—totalling about 93,000 miles (150,000 km) in length—distribute oxygen and nutrients to all living tissues in the body.

## The blood vessels

With a single exception—the pulmonary arteries—the veins and arteries are distinguished by function: arteries carry oxygen-rich blood away from the heart to the body tissues; veins return oxygen-depleted blood to the heart, where the pulmonary arteries send it to the lungs to be recharged with oxygen. Both have the same general form and structure.

Surrounding a central channel, the **lumen**, blood vessels are made up of three layers. The innermost, the **tunica intima**, is a lining composed of endothelium, only one cell thick, and supporting elastic fibres. Endothelial cells are flat, scalelike (hence termed "squamous"), and smooth—blood flows across the inside surface with a minimum of disturbance. A thicker, middle layer, the **tunica media**, is made up of smooth muscle and some elastic tissue. Contraction or dilation of vessel walls can raise or lower the blood pressure. The external layer, the **tunica adventitia**, is composed of collagen fibres, which give the vessel toughness.

Although the heart's action delivers force in discrete impulses, blood flow is smooth and continuous owing to an elastic rebound in vessel walls: vessels bulge somewhat with the rush of blood during the heart's stroke (systole), but return elastically to shape between strokes (diastole), thus pushing blood onward in an uninterrupted rush. Pressure is higher nearer the origin of the impulse and lower at longer distances, as friction in the system—in this case passage through miles of blood vessels—slows the fluid. Arteries, thus, must withstand higher pressures than veins, and therefore have thicker walls than veins, in which the tunica media is considerably thinner.

The main arteries leaving the heart branch into smaller arteries, and into still smaller arteries and then—within an organ or other tissue—into thin-walled arterioles, with diameters of about $1/100$ in (0.3 mm). Arterioles further divide into a meshwork of smaller channels called capillaries, which are so narrow (on the order of $3/10,000$ in, or 0.008 mm) that red blood cells are just able to pass through them, one at a time. Capillaries make up a fine net, a capillary bed, which is the endpoint of oxygenated circulation. From the capillaries, blood drains into vessels that return it to the heart and into venules, which join to form successively larger veins leading towards the heart. Because pressure is so much lower in the return side of the system, veins have valves spaced along their inner surfaces that allow blood to pass in the heartward direction but not back.

Capillary walls consist of endothelium only, one cell thick, which allows oxygen and nutrients to pass through, into the interstitial fluid around adjoining tissues. The endothelium also ensures that cellular waste products are expelled into the circulation, for eventual disposal by various organs.

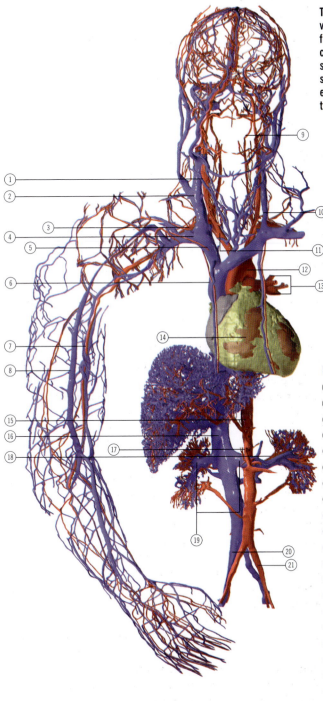

The heart and a part of the venous system; shown here, from the front, is the return circulation on the upper right side—all draining into the superior vena cava—and the extensive vascular branchings of the liver.

**Key**

1. Common carotid artery
2. Internal jugular vein
3. Right subclavian artery
4. Right subclavian vein
5. Brachiocephalic vein
6. Superior vena cava
7. Brachial artery
8. Cephalic vein
9. External carotid artery
10. Internal jugular
11. Brachiocephalic artery
12. Aortic arch
13. Pulmonary arteries
14. Heart
15. Abdominal aorta
16. Inferior vena cava
17. Coeliac trunk
18. Renal artery
19. Renal veins
20. Common iliac vein
21. Common iliac artery

# THE ARTERIAL SYSTEM

A NETWORK OF ARTERIES DISTRIBUTES NUTRIENTS and oxygenated blood throughout the body. An additional, shorter pathway, the pulmonary circuit, delivers oxygen-depleted blood to the lungs.

## The heart

Oxygenated blood is brought to the left chambers of the heart, from the lungs, by several pulmonary veins, which merge into two vessels converging at the left atrium. With the help of the atrium, the left ventricle pushes oxygen-rich blood into the aorta. It leaves the heart directed upward, but quickly curves through a full half-circle, the aortic arch, to descend through the trunk. Projecting upward from the top of the aortic arch, three arteries branch to the shoulders, arms, and head: the brachiocephalic trunk (also called the innominate artery), left common carotid, and left subclavian arteries. Here, as in the trunk and head, there is a slight asymmetry: carotid and subclavian on the left side spring individually from the aorta; on the right side they branch subsequently from the brachiocephalic trunk. The first arteries to divide from the aorta, however, arise at the base of the ascending aorta, just as it leaves the heart; these are the left and right coronary arteries, which supply the heart muscle with oxygen-rich blood.

## The head

The left and right carotid and vertebral arteries bring blood to the head. The carotids divide into two main branches, the internal and external, which supply the face, skull, scalp, upper neck, eyes, ears, and much of the cerebrum. The vertebral arteries, the first and largest branchings from the subclavian arteries, run together at the base of the skull to form the basilar artery, which sends blood through its branches to the cerebellum, midbrain, and parts of the cerebrum, mostly at the back. Other branches of the vertebral arteries also reach into the cerebellum, as well as running to the spine.

## The trunk

Housing most of the body's central organs, the trunk receives blood through aortic branches directed at maintaining organ function, but also branching to supply muscle, nerve, bone, and skin in the same region. The descending aorta's upper segment is called the thoracic aorta; it supplies the lungs, oesophagus, and pericardium. Its lower segment, before it divides into branches to the lower limbs, is the abdominal aorta; its first principal branches—arising from an enlarged offshoot called the coeliac trunk—are the common hepatic, splenic, and left gastric arteries. Below the coeliac trunk are the superior mesenteric, renal, and inferior mesenteric. At about the level of the umbilicus, the aorta divides into the two common iliac arteries, which redivide into internal and external branches, supplying pelvic organs and muscles. The larger external iliac becomes the femoral artery as it descends into the thigh.

## The limbs

Arterial networks serving muscles and other tissue of the arm arise from continuations of the subclavian artery, chiefly the axillary and brachial arteries (to the radial and ulnar arteries). In the leg, the femoral artery and its main branches—the deep femoral and popliteal (to the anterior and posterior tibial, and peroneal arteries)—provide blood supply.

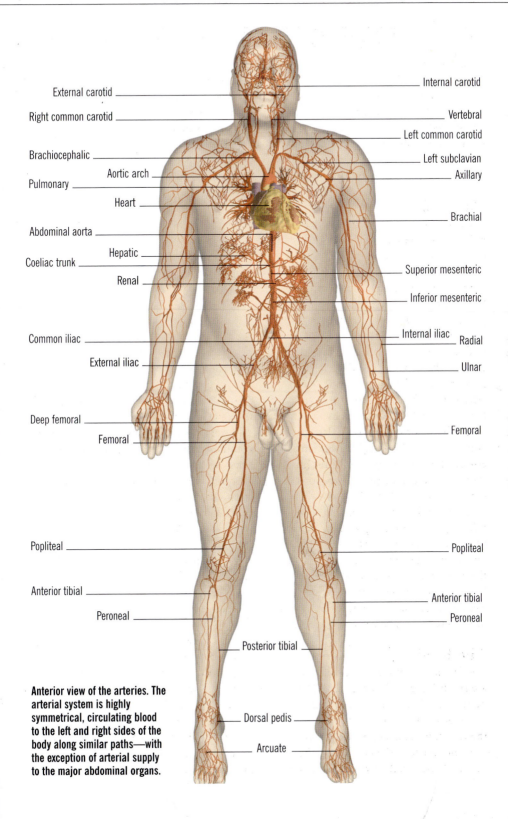

External carotid

Right common carotid

Brachiocephalic

Aortic arch

Pulmonary

Heart

Abdominal aorta

Hepatic

Coeliac trunk

Renal

Common iliac

External iliac

Deep femoral

Femoral

Popliteal

Anterior tibial

Peroneal

Internal carotid

Vertebral

Left common carotid

Left subclavian

Axillary

Brachial

Superior mesenteric

Inferior mesenteric

Internal iliac

Radial

Ulnar

Femoral

Popliteal

Anterior tibial

Peroneal

Posterior tibial

Dorsal pedis

Arcuate

**Anterior view of the arteries. The arterial system is highly symmetrical, circulating blood to the left and right sides of the body along similar paths—with the exception of arterial supply to the major abdominal organs.**

# THE VENOUS SYSTEM

INTERSTITIAL FLUID SURROUNDING THE BODY'S CELLS makes available a constantly renewed source of oxygen and nutrients; it also accumulates cellular waste material, including carbon dioxide. In the capillary beds, these metabolic products pass into the blood, and from there into venules, then into larger returning streams, the veins, towards the heart. Blood in the venous system is, thus, in a sense "spent". It has lost a good deal of its propelling pressure, needs recharging with oxygen, and may carry a burden of raw nutrients as well as the ordinary byproducts of cellular activity.

## The veins

The venous side of the circulatory system consists of thinner-walled vessels than arteries, though veins are usually somewhat larger in channel diameter, or **lumen**. Because veins conduct fluid at a lower pressure than do arteries, vein walls need not be as strong. To lessen the effort needed to return blood to the chest, many veins have several one-way valves along their lengths (very small and very large veins, such as the brachiocephalic and pulmonary veins, have no valves). These valves are flexible, pouchy endothelial structures (up to three per valve) found in the vein wall; they are pursed tightly by backward flow and close the vein to any surge in that direction.

The major veins occur more or less as matching return loops with the major arteries and usually bear matching names: a femoral vein, and its tributary venules, drains the capillary beds and arteriole network supplied by the femoral artery, and so forth. Exceptions, however, are not uncommon: blood from the head is returned by the jugular veins (not by "carotid" veins). Also, more major veins than major arteries appear to run through the limbs. In the limbs, generally, blood is supplied deep to the tissues and works through capillary beds towards the surface, where it must be collected over a wider area, from many superficial veins. Thus, in the leg, the great saphenous vein (the longest vein in the body) and small saphenous vein have no exact arterial counterparts or corresponding names.

The veins eventually converge at the right atrium of the heart in two main trunk veins: the superior and inferior vena cava. Blood is pushed onward by the right ventricle, through the pulmonary arteries and lungs, and directly then to the left side of the heart through the pulmonary veins. The distinction between vein and artery is always in relation to the direction of blood flow: oxygenated blood flows in the pulmonary veins, *towards* the heart (its left side) and oxygen-poor blood flows in the pulmonary arteries, *away* from the heart (its right side).

## Portal circulation

When blood is collected and carried by vessels from one capillary bed to another before being returned to the heart, the intervening circulation is called portal. Most commonly this refers to circulation between the gastrointestinal tract (and spleen) and liver—through the portal vein. Blood that has recently absorbed a heavy load of nutrients, and perhaps some toxins, from digestive processes cannot circulate without first being processed in the liver, through its dense meshwork of venules and capillaries. Leaving the liver, blood flows via the hepatic veins directly into the inferior vena cava.

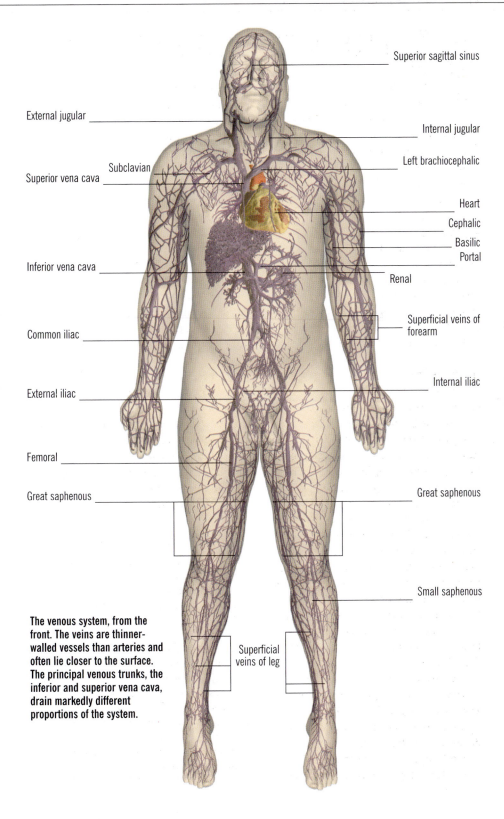

Superior sagittal sinus

External jugular

Internal jugular

Left brachiocephalic

Subclavian

Superior vena cava

Heart

Cephalic

Basilic

Portal

Inferior vena cava

Renal

Common iliac

Superficial veins of forearm

External iliac

Internal iliac

Femoral

Great saphenous

Great saphenous

Small saphenous

**The venous system, from the front. The veins are thinner-walled vessels than arteries and often lie closer to the surface. The principal venous trunks, the inferior and superior vena cava, drain markedly different proportions of the system.**

Superficial veins of leg

# OUR LIFE'S BLOOD

BLOOD, THE LIFE-GIVING LIQUID THAT circulates throughout the body, is a living tissue—its complex cellular constituents just happen to be mobile instead of fixed within a fibrous or bony framework.

As well as oxygen, the blood absorbs or distributes a large number of substances that require transport around the body: nutrients, proteins, metabolic byproducts, hormones, and, unfortunately, pathogens. Blood also has an important role to play in temperature regulation, taking heat up and conducting it within and around the body, or closer to the surface for cooling.

## Blood makeup

The volume of blood in an average adult lies in the range of 8–10 pints (4–5 litres) for a female, and 10–12 pints (5–6 litres) for a male. About 55 percent of it is plasma, a clear and slightly yellowish fluid, which is mostly water in which are dissolved over 100 substances including nutrients, hormones, antibodies, and waste substances.

The composition of blood constantly changes as substances enter or leave the bloodstream; various **homeostatic** mechanisms—mostly parts of the endocrine system—monitor and control certain basic blood properties, maintaining proper volume, density, pH, and chemical reactivity. Any serious disturbance, for example, of blood's osmotic potential, might cause **interstitial fluid** to be pulled into the circulation with consequent injury to cells. A continual balance among ions—principally of sodium, but also potassium, calcium, and phosphate—is achieved through several fine-control mechanisms.

## Blood clotting

Platelets, or thrombocytes, operate in blood clotting: they stick together immediately at the site of a wound but also stage the clotting process with the aid of plasma components such as calcium, and several proteins and enzymes that are together known as clotting factors. In clotting, a plasma protein, **fibrinogen**, is altered (**to fibrin**) and formed into a barricade net across the site of injury. Platelets are shed in great numbers from large parent cells in the marrow; about a billion are circulating at any time.

## Blood cells

The remaining 45 percent of blood consists of two distinct cell types—red and white—plus platelets. Of the three, only the white cells (leucocytes) possess nuclei within their cellular envelopes. The red blood cells (erythrocytes) carry oxygen; trillions of red cells circulate at any one time and they make up 99 percent of the blood cell population. Within the red cells are large proteins, **haemoglobin**, that attach oxygen where concentration is high and release it where oxygen presence is low.

White blood cells identify and attack invading pathogens (but may also be stirred by false alarms, causing hypersensitivity reactions). There are three kinds of white blood cells, and several subtypes of each:

- **granulocytes**: these cells are active against pathogens, both detecting and destroying cells that are sensed to be alien or defective in some way.
- **monocytes**: they are the largest of the white cells and the least numerous, making up 3–6 percent of all leucocytes. They are voracious; after

engulfing a suspect intruder, they can also trigger a lymphocyte response. Monocytes circulate in the blood and lymph, but the **macrophage** (so-called "big eater") variety migrates into tissues.

- **lymphocytes**: these are of two major types, T-cells and B-cells, present both in blood and lymph. A third type, NK ("natural killer"), is also often distinguished, as its origin and action differ from T-cell types. B-cells produce large protein molecules called **antibodies**, which are patterned to disable specific pathogens—hence B-cells are the key element in what is termed "specific immunity". (A group of about 20 circulating proteins,

collectively called complement, assist in destruction after an antibody has attached itself to its target.) T-cells destroy pathogens, but also modulate the immune system's response, activating or deactivating B-cells and other T-cells. NK cells identify possible targets differently, which makes them more successful than other types against threats such as viruses or tumour cells—where the cause of concern may lie inside a cell that is outwardly normal enough to pass lymphocyte scrutiny.

On average, red blood cells survive for about 120 days, so replacement is a continuing activity in the bone marrow.

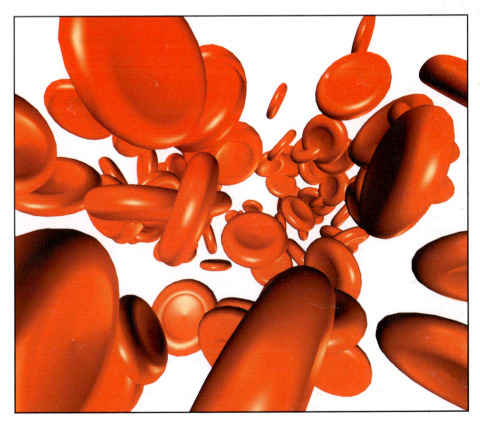

# THE HEART

THE DESIGN OF THE HEART MAY be likened to a pair of two-stage pumps side by side within a shared housing. The housing, however, consists almost entirely of cardiac muscle—with patches of fibrous tissue filling out parts of its shape—and its sequenced contractions squeeze blood into the aorta at a rate of 1–2 gallons (4–8 litres) per minute. It works continuously, too: 100,000 beats a day, over two and a half billion in an average life.

The interior of the heart is divided into similar halves, each with two chambers, the atrium and ventricle. The right and left ventricles are separated by a muscular dividing wall, the septum. A tough double-layered protective sac, called the pericardium, envelops the entire muscle. Between the layers is a smooth endothelial lining and a small amount of fluid within that space, which reduces friction and somewhat dampens the effects of constant heart motion.

## The heart rate

The two atria assist the ventricles only, quickly and forcibly filling them for the main ventricular pumping stroke to follow. These steps are called **atrial systole** (atrial contraction) and **ventricular systole** (ventricular contraction). The interval between is the **diastole**.

Coordination of the systoles and regulation of their rate is accomplished through electrical means. In the wall of the right atrium is a concentration of special, fast-contracting muscle fibres

**The heart, seen from behind, is connected to an array of supply and return vessels. Oxygenated blood leaves by the aorta; depleted blood returns by the inferior and superior vena cava (behind other vessels).**

Left subclavian artery

Descending aorta

Left pulmonary artery

Left atrium

Left pulmonary veins

Coronary sinus

Left ventricle

Apex of heart

Left common carotid artery

Brachiocephalic trunk

Arch of aorta

Ascending aorta

Superior vena cava

Right pulmonary artery

Right pulmonary veins

Right atrium

Inferior vena cava

collectively known as the **sinoatrial (SA) node**. Their action initiates a spreading wave of electrical breakdown and contraction across the atrial muscle. The impulse is halted for about a tenth of a second at the atrioventricular (AV) node, before continuing—through specially conductive fibres called the His bundle—to excite ventricular contraction. The SA node is often referred to as the heart's pacemaker; its internal cycle of electrical buildup and discharge repeats in a rhythmic, automatic way about every eight-tenths of a second (at rest).

Speeding up or slowing down the rate of contraction cycles is brought about through the autonomic nervous system. Centres in the medulla oblongata sense changes in blood pressure and its chemical properties. The **cardioacceleratory centre** responds by sending signals through sympathetic fibres to accelerate the heart rate; the **cardioinhibitory centre** acts through parasympathetic fibres to slow it down. Both work on the SA node by altering electrochemically the time needed for firing and recovery in a cycle.

## The heart valves

The ventricles can be shut off from the atria, or from the blood vessels at their other ends, by sets of two valves. Passage between the atria and ventricles is controlled by **atrioventricular valves**: the **tricuspid valve** on the right and the mitral valve on the left. At the ventricular exits are the pulmonary valve and the aortic valve, collectively termed the **semilunar valves**. Other valves, much less developed, guard the atrial entrances (except at the superior vena cava).

In this anterior cutaway view, the heart's chambers and valves are exposed.

Brachiocephalic trunk

Ascending aorta

Superior vena cava

Ascending aorta

Right atrium

Tricuspid valve

Cordae tendineae

Papillary muscle

Inferior vena cava

Left common carotid artery

Left subclavian artery

Arch of the aorta

Pulmonary trunk

Left pulmonary artery

Left atrium

Aortic semilunar valve

Mitral valve

Left ventricle

Interventricular septum

Right ventricle

# THE LYMPHATIC SYSTEM

PERMEATING THE BODY TISSUES IS A second network of fluid-filled vessels, the lymphatic system. It augments the body's vascular system in respect of two functions: by collecting excess fluid and waste from the tissues, and by destroying any intruding or unfamiliar cells.

Most lymphatic activity takes place in numerous swellings called lymph nodes, found astride lymphatic channels and their junctions. The main lymph organs are the spleen and thymus (which begins to atrophy in adolescence, gradually becoming fatty tissue). The tonsils are mostly composed of lymphatic tissue, too, and tend to shrink or even disappear with age.

## One-way flow

Lymph vessels, unlike blood vessels, do not form circulatory loops; they terminate at their capillary endpoints. There is no single pump, such as the heart, to cause flow. Lymph vessels do, however, possess interior valves—much like those of blood veins—so that contractions of nearby muscles tend to squeeze fluid through vessels in the direction favoured by the valves. This direction is always away from the tissue beds and towards larger and larger lymphatic channels and trunks, which ultimately drain into the left and right subclavian veins by way of two lymphatic ducts.

Such a pumping mechanism, albeit somewhat fitful and sluggish, moves fluid away from tissues; the supply of fluid is that which normally infiltrates the spaces around the cells (**interstitial fluid**), which is also taken up by the general venous circulation. However, about a sixth of this volume actually ends up in lymph channels instead.

The lymph network is not symmetrical: a far larger region drains into the left side duct, the thoracic duct, than drains into the right lymphatic duct. All of the vessels and nodes of the lower body, including an especially rich supply of vessels around the intestines, contribute to a convergence called the cisterna chyli, which is the origin of the thoracic duct. Vessels emptying into the right lymphatic duct serve the right arm, the thorax, and the head.

## Immune function

Within the lymph system, macrophages and lymphocytes are exposed to material flushed from tissues. Pathogenic organisms, cellular debris, or defective cells (including potentially cancerous cells) excite a reaction that generally results in their destruction.

The lymph nodes are not merely enlarged junctions; they have a structural capsule, with internal dividers and a fibrous net, which hold in place nodules formed from dense clumps of **lymphocytes**. Lymph traverses the node through a maze of channels lying between the nodules. Here, B-cells, in particular, are present in large numbers, as well as other lymphocytes.

**Macrophages**, which do not have the very specific appetites of B-cells, engulf anything that seems out of place. When levels of activity rise within a node—in the presence of a recognized pathogen—new lymphocytes and **antibodies** are produced, and the result may be manifested as swelling and soreness in that area.

# The spleen

The spleen is one of the major "housekeeping" organs and the largest lymphatic organ. It is draped by the diaphragm, nestling to the rear against the lower ribs on the left side. The spleen has significant immune system functions and removes worn out red blood cells from the circulation, recycling some components and disposing of other cellular debris.

A fibrous capsule encloses the spleen and sends strands into the interior to support its tissues. A **hilum** (a hollow) on the spleen's underside receives its blood vessels, the splenic artery and splenic vein. Splenic tissues are of two main types: patchy nodes of white pulp, surrounded by red pulp.

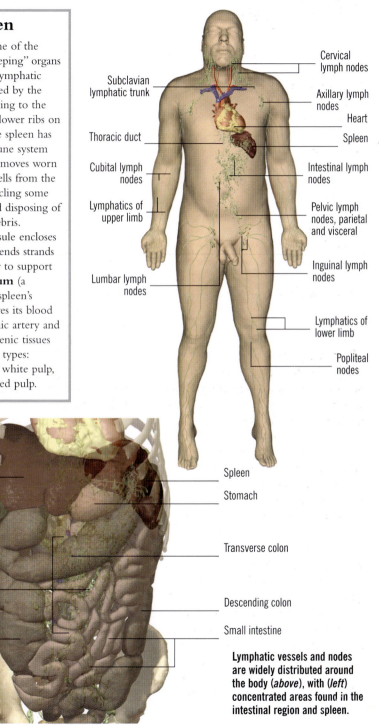

Cervical lymph nodes

Subclavian lymphatic trunk

Axillary lymph nodes

Heart

Thoracic duct

Spleen

Cubital lymph nodes

Intestinal lymph nodes

Lymphatics of upper limb

Pelvic lymph nodes, parietal and visceral

Inguinal lymph nodes

Lumbar lymph nodes

Lymphatics of lower limb

Popliteal nodes

Liver

Spleen

Stomach

Gallbladder

Transverse colon

Intestinal lymph nodes

Descending colon

Ascending colon

Small intestine

**Lymphatic vessels and nodes are widely distributed around the body (*above*), with (*left*) concentrated areas found in the intestinal region and spleen.**

# THE RESPIRATORY SYSTEM

THE CHIEF FORM OF ENERGY PRODUCTION in the body—that is, its method of burning its stores of fuel—is aerobic **metabolism**, a process that utilizes oxygen and produces carbon dioxide as waste. When someone breathes, special membranes in the person's lungs absorb oxygen from the air, while at the same time releasing carbon dioxide into the atmosphere.

The complete apparatus for exchanging these two gases in the blood, the respiratory system, consists of airways—called the respiratory tract—and the lungs themselves. Larger components of the respiratory tract include the nose, mouth, throat, and trachea (the windpipe). At its lower end, the trachea divides into two major passageways, the bronchi, that enter the left and right lobar clusters of the lungs.

In the course of ventilation, oxygen enters into the blood circulation by a process of **diffusion**, passing across the lung membranes until relative pressures of the gas approach balance on both sides of the exceedingly thin alveolar wall between blood and air. Carbon dioxide, meanwhile, bubbles out of the blood, crossing the membrane in the opposite direction.

Rhythmic filling and expulsion of air, breathing, takes place (at rest) about 12–16 times per minute, or an average of 20,000 times per day.

## Breathing

The space inside the thoracic "cage" formed by the ribs, sternum, and backbone is mainly occupied by the lungs. These are grouped into lobes, three on the right and two on the left (accommodating the mass of the heart). Each group is surrounded by and attached to a protective sac called the visceral **pleura**.

Another pleural coating, the parietal layer, lines all the inner thoracic surfaces of the cage, with attachment to the ribs, vertebrae, sternum, and pericardium. Fluid produced by the pleural tissue fills the spaces between the two layers. The floor of the thoracic cavity—and that which divides the thoracic and abdominal cavities—is the diaphragm, a thin sheet of muscle and fibre. The diaphragm is the chief muscle used in breathing.

## The diaphragm

When relaxed, the diaphragm bulges loosely upward, like a dome, over the packed abdominal organs beneath it. As it contracts it pushes these organs down, creating space in the thoracic cavity. At the same time, external intercostal muscles lift the ribs upward and outward. The atmospheric pressure of air expands the lungs to fill the enlarged thoracic volume. Normally, as these muscles relax, the chest and abdomen sag back into place, pushing air out of the lungs. The internal intercostal muscles, which pull the ribs together, can assist, or actively expel air in forced breathing.

Anterior view of the airways and lungs. The diaphragm, which is draped over the upper abdominal organs, pushes downward on them, allowing the lungs above to expand.

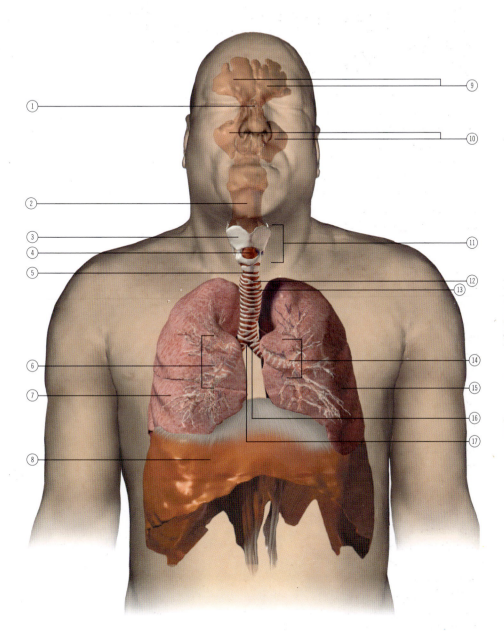

**Key**

1. Ethmoid sinus
2. Pharynx
3. Thyroid cartilage
4. Medial cricothyroid ligament
5. Tracheal cartilage
6. Right bronchial tree
7. Right lung
8. Diaphragm
9. Frontal sinuses
10. Maxillary sinuses
11. Larynx
12. Trachea
13. Annular ligament of trachea
14. Left bronchial tree
15. Left lung
16. Left primary bronchus
17. Tracheal bifurcation

# THE MOUTH, NOSE, AND THROAT

THE RESPIRATORY TRACT, THE AIRWAY THAT provides passage to the lungs, includes the nose, the mouth, the pharynx (throat), the larynx (upper trachea), and the trachea (windpipe). Along this course, inspired (that is, breathed-in) air is moistened, warmed, and filtered before reaching the lungs.

Air normally enters through the nose, where nostril hairs filter out coarser airborne particles. Before passing to the pharynx, incoming air is swirled through a spiral labyrinth formed by several curved platy conchoid bones—the nasal turbinates. These open onto membrane-lined cavities in the bones—the paranasal sinuses—which warm and moisten the air.

The inner surfaces all along the airway, and in the sinuses, moisten themselves with a sticky mucus that absorbs the finer air particles, including airborne organisms such as bacteria and viruses. Mucus also humidifies air. Air taken in through the mouth does not undergo nasal filtration, nor is it likely to be equally moisturized or warmed.

Mucous membranes in the nose, sinuses, larynx, and trachea are covered in microscopic hairlike projections called **cilia**. The cilia sway in slow, rhythmic waves to move mucus, bearing its burden of extracted particles, towards the throat, in order that it may be swallowed—then disposed of through normal digestive processes.

## The larynx and vocal cords

The segment of the airway between the pharynx and trachea, the larynx, is a tube formed of cartilages pieced into shape by ligaments and connective membranes. Two sharp folds—the vocal cords—opposite one another in the surface membranes run back to front across the laryngeal passage. When not in use they lie back loosely against the sides of the passageway. Muscles attached to the folds can pull the folds taut and inward, constricting the passage so that air expelled through them sets up vibrations—the amplitude and frequencies depend on the force of the air and the tension with which the muscles stretch the vocal folds. Sounds produced in this way are amplified and affected by resonances in the throat, mouth, nose, and sinuses.

The vocal folds lengthen in the natural course of growth, causing the voice's pitch to fall—most dramatically during the male teenage growth spurt.

Tensing the vocal cords is accomplished by the cricothyroid muscle; several muscles relax them or help control tension during the production of sound (principally the vocalis, a part of the thyroarytenoid muscle).

The largest laryngeal cartilage, the thyroid cartilage, comprises two plates that meet at an angle right in the front of the throat. These form, in males, the external Adam's apple, as they join at a sharper, outwardly jutting angle than in females.

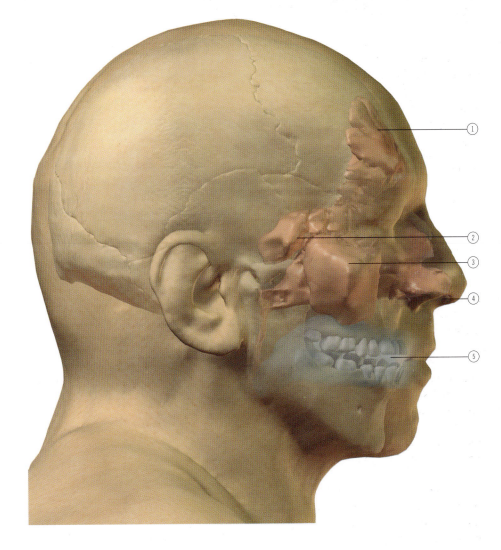

**Key**

① Frontal sinus
② Sphenoid sinus
③ Maxillary sinus
④ Nasal vestibule
⑤ Oral cavity

The sinus cavities have important functions: they help moisturize inspired air and also trap dust and pathogens. As resonant spaces, they provide individual voices with much of their sound quality.

# THE LUNGS

THE LEFT AND RIGHT PRIMARY BRONCHI entering the lungs divide many times into smaller bronchi—often referred to as successive "generations"—and then into even narrower bronchioles, the ultimate offshoots of which have diameters of about ⁵⁄₁₀₀ in (1 mm) or less. The entire network is sometimes visualized as a "bronchial tree". The bronchial walls are made of cartilage, with a good deal of elastic fibre, and are underlain by intersecting strands of

muscle. The interior has a constantly moist mucosal layer. In the bronchioles, the cartilage is absent and muscle fibre scant; instead, collagen with some elastic reinforcement comprises most of the wall.

The bronchioles terminate in tiny air-exchange globules called alveolar sacs. These hang like clusters of grapes at the

**The lungs, from the front, envelope the heart and major vessels, though all direct contact is through the endothelial lining surfaces (the pleura and pericardium).**

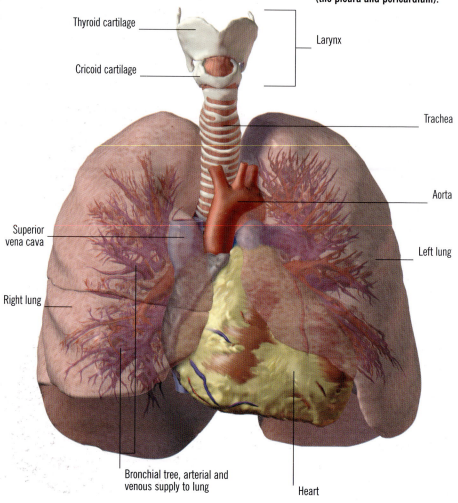

Thyroid cartilage

Cricoid cartilage

Larynx

Trachea

Aorta

Superior
vena cava

Left lung

Right lung

Bronchial tree, arterial and
venous supply to lung

Heart

end of the smallest bronchioles. Inside each are short tubes, alveolar ducts, which give access to bunched pouchings called alveoli. There are about 300 million alveoli in the lungs, presenting a total working surface of approximately 750 square feet (70 square meters).

Capillary beds surround the alveoli, exposing oxygen-depleted blood to inspired air across a membrane wall that is only 40-millionths of an inch thick (0.001 mm). A fluid film coating the inner surfaces of the alveoli dissolves oxygen and hastens its diffusion across the thin barrier between the blood and the atmosphere. Oxygen makes up 21 percent of air; its presence in alveolar air normally drops to about 15 percent—in other words, the alveoli are efficient enough to remove a quarter of the oxygen from the air. In the exchange, blood that enters the lungs is, typically, 75–80 percent oxygen-saturated (that is, as a percentage of all the oxygen it could carry); it leaves the lungs 94–98 percent saturated. Carbon dioxide, at the same time, diffuses outward across the alveolar membrane at a nearly equal rate. The body's **homeostatic** processes actually work to keep blood carbon dioxide levels constant by controlling the breathing reflex; regulation of blood oxygen follows as a consequence.

# Respiratory development

Breathing does not take place in the womb. The fetus's need for oxygen is satisfied by the mother's blood supply—oxygen is extracted by the **placenta** and circulated to fetal tissues. From the time the lungs begin to form until shortly before birth, they are filled with fluid and are not a source of oxygen, although intermittent breathing actions do take place as part of fetal development. By the time the baby emerges, the lungs have been drained and are functional, though a newborn infant will not try to use them until the placental supply has been cut. Once cut, carbon dioxide levels rise, triggering the autonomic breathing reflex in the brain and bringing the breathing muscles and lungs into action.

**Back view: circulation through the lungs is from the pulmonary arteries and out through the pulmonary veins (below the pulmonary arteries). The 16–20 cartilage rings that make up the trachea do not extend all the way around; smooth muscle and connective fibre complete the rings at the back.**

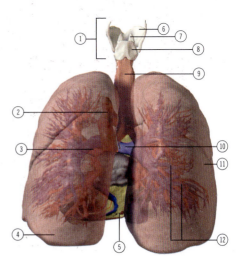

## Key

1. Larynx
2. Aorta
3. Left pulmonary artery
4. Left lung
5. Heart
6. Thyroid cartilage
7. Arytenoid cartilage
8. Cricoid cartilage
9. Trachea
10. Right pulmonary vein
11. Right lung
12. Bronchial tree, arterial and venous supply to lung

# THE DIGESTIVE SYSTEM

THE BODY NORMALLY OBTAINS NOURISHMENT THROUGH a process that starts and finishes along the alimentary canal, which runs from the mouth to the anus. Its component segments—the mouth, throat (pharynx), oesophagus, stomach, small and large intestines—are sites of distinct digestive activities, assisted or carried out by other organs collectively termed the accessory digestive organs. These include the teeth, tongue, liver, gallbladder, and pancreas.

Several accessory organs have other functions, too: the pancreas controls blood sugar levels, and the liver has a great many functions, including sorting and processing nutrients once absorbed from the alimentary canal. The gallbladder, however, functions only as a digestive accessory, collecting and releasing bile to make fats soluble for digestion.

The walls enclosing the alimentary canal are coated in muscle that consists typically of two smooth-muscle layers. The stomach, which performs vigorous muscular work on ingested food, has a third layer, an innermost ply of oblique muscle. Smooth muscles are not consciously controlled; their activity is regulated by the autonomic nervous system and by hormones.

Slow, coordinated waves of contraction ripple along the alimentary walls, always pushing digestive contents towards the far end, the anus. This continual undulatory action, called **peristalsis**, may occasionally become stronger along some stretches of the canal, as after a meal or in defecating.

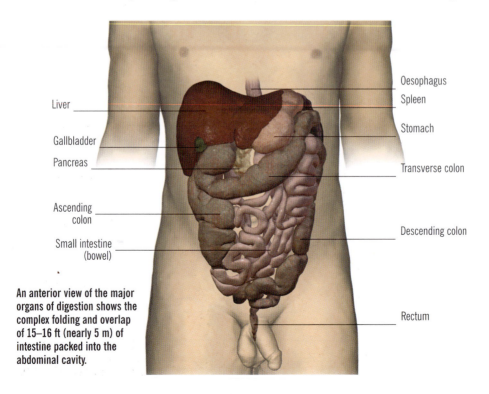

Liver

Gallbladder

Pancreas

Ascending colon

Small intestine (bowel)

Oesophagus

Spleen

Stomach

Transverse colon

Descending colon

Rectum

An anterior view of the major organs of digestion shows the complex folding and overlap of 15–16 ft (nearly 5 m) of intestine packed into the abdominal cavity.

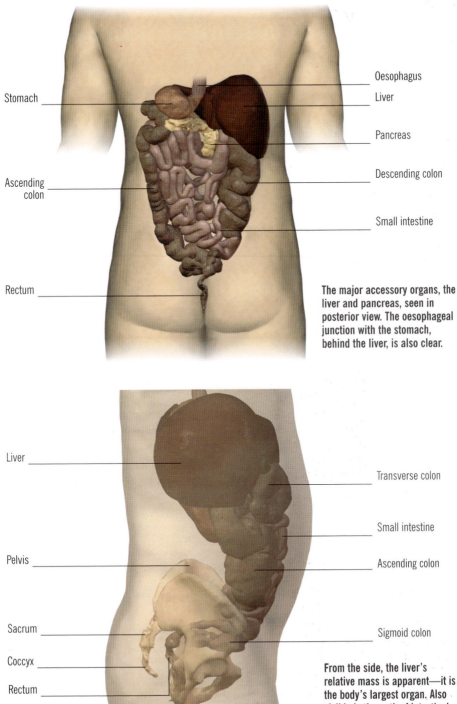

Stomach

Oesophagus

Liver

Pancreas

Descending colon

Ascending
colon

Small intestine

Rectum

The major accessory organs, the
liver and pancreas, seen in
posterior view. The oesophageal
junction with the stomach,
behind the liver, is also clear.

Liver

Transverse colon

Small intestine

Pelvis

Ascending colon

Sacrum

Sigmoid colon

Coccyx

Rectum

From the side, the liver's
relative mass is apparent—it is
the body's largest organ. Also
visible is the path of intestinal
descent through the pelvic floor.

# HOW THE DIGESTIVE SYSTEM WORKS

IN A VERY GENERAL WAY, WE refer to substances with nutritional value as "food", but natural forms, such as vegetables, meats, grains, etc., are seldom of immediate use to the body. Before food can be transmuted into energy or new body tissue it must undergo considerable physical and chemical change, which is accomplished in the digestive system.

## Food and enzymes

Useful substances in food (including water, of course) may be categorized roughly as carbohydrates, fats, proteins, vitamins, minerals, and fibre.

- Carbohydrates—starch and sugar—are fuel; they are broken down by **enzymes** into simple sugars for **metabolic** needs or linked into special storage forms.
- Fats, also a source and store of energy, may be transformed in many ways and incorporated into substances necessary for the building and function of cells.
- The very numerous ingested proteins are split by enzymes into their component amino acids (20 of which are used by the body). These are then available for reassembly into new enzyme or cell proteins, or for gluconeogenesis, another pathway for energy production.
- Vitamins and minerals, substances that are not produced in the body, are chemically necessary to many metabolic activities. Minerals such as calcium and iron are also essential for tissue (bone and blood) formation.
- Fibre, composed of vegetal cellulose, cannot be digested, but it gives bulk and cohesion to intestinal waste, assisting its physical transport through the system.

## Digestive enzymes

Enzymes are biological **catalysts**; they chemically alter certain substances without themselves becoming altered. Their presence causes specific reactions to take place far more rapidly than would otherwise happen—rates may be accelerated by a factor of thousands or even millions.

Enzymes possess molecular shapes that fit, in a highly specific way, some part of another molecule, a target molecule called the **substrate** of a particular enzyme. The substrate molecule is held in an enzyme's fitted region (its active site) and a stressed substrate bond breaks. Pieces of the split substrate, the enzyme products, detach themselves, perhaps to be absorbed or to be further reduced by different enzymes. The enzyme, meanwhile, is unchanged and free to lock onto new substrate.

**Intracellular** enzymes work inside cells; they speed up metabolic reactions. **Extracellular** enzymes, operating outside cells, include those active in digestion. Digestive enzymes—secreted in the salivary glands, stomach, pancreas, and small intestine—have in common a chemical result that breaks bonds by allowing water ions to attach at a substrate's snipped ends. This reaction between substrate and water, called **hydrolysis** ("water splitting"), is greatly facilitated by an enzyme's deforming effect on a particular bond.

Digestion often involves a sequence of actions by different enzymes, as for example with starch: the salivary enzyme **amylase** first cuts off double-sugars (maltose) that are then reduced to a simple sugar (glucose) by the pancreatic enzyme **maltase**.

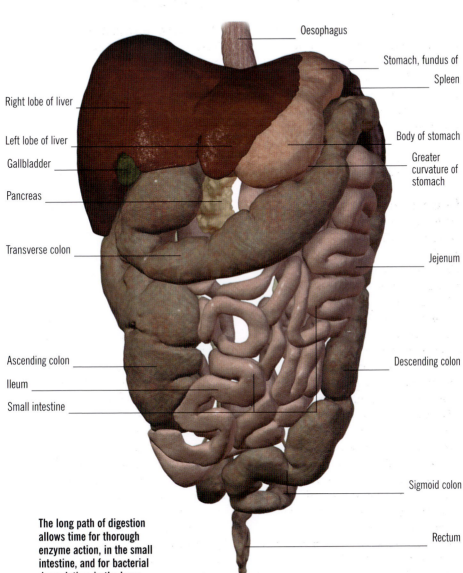

Oesophagus

Stomach, fundus of

Spleen

Right lobe of liver

Left lobe of liver

Gallbladder

Pancreas

Body of stomach

Greater curvature of stomach

Transverse colon

Jejenum

Ascending colon

Ileum

Small intestine

Descending colon

Sigmoid colon

Rectum

The long path of digestion allows time for thorough enzyme action, in the small intestine, and for bacterial degradation, in the large intestine. If, as in disease, passage is significantly speeded up, inadequate nutrients are absorbed.

# THE MOUTH AND THROAT

DIGESTION BEGINS IN THE MOUTH. HERE, teeth tear and mash food; saliva moistens it and initiates breakdown by **enzymes**; and the tongue mixes everything, at the same time providing evaluative sensations—tastes—of the digestive system's intake.

## The teeth

Adults have 32 teeth, 16 in each jaw. Differently shaped teeth accomplish different tasks as part of the pulping process: the jaw's four sharp incisors, at the very front, cut food; its two canines grip and pierce it; at the rear, four premolars and six molars perform thorough grinding and crushing.

Although they seem somewhat bonelike and they are firmly socketed in bone, teeth actually develop from a different line of cells, odontoblasts and ameloblasts, that have highly mineralized coats, dentin and enamel. A tooth's interior, the pulp, is living tissue with blood and a nerve supply. Its outermost layer, the enamel, is the hardest substance produced by living organisms.

## The chewing process

Chewing is powered chiefly by the masseter and temporalis muscles, which lift the mandible (lower jaw) against the opposing maxillary surface. Cheek muscles assist by pressing food back into the mouth cavity as it is forced to the sides by molar action.

The mouth's enclosed volume is created, in the front, by closed lips; at the top, by the hard and soft palates; its floor is the tongue. At the rear, the pharynx (throat) receives food when the tongue pushes a chewed portion, a bolus, back into the throat's entrance. When food touches the throat's back and sides, it initiates the coordinated reflex called swallowing.

As a bolus reaches the throat, constrictor muscles squeeze the food downward towards the oesophagus; other muscles lift the larynx upward slightly, at the same time pulling a cartilaginous flap, the epiglottis, across the entrance to the airway. The epiglottis, covered in mucous membrane, seats itself snugly against the back of the tongue, at its lowest part, and prevents food from being aspirated, or "going down the wrong way". After a bolus has passed, the muscles relax; the larynx falls back into place, dropping the epiglottis away from the tongue and reopening the airway.

## The salivary glands

There are three pairs of main salivary glands and numerous minor, or accessory, glands. The salivary glands secrete a mucous liquid, the consistency and makeup of which is variable. Along with water, mucus, and miscellaneous salts and proteins, saliva contains enzymes that begin the digestive process even as food is still being chewed. Amylase, which is responsible for breaking down starch, is its principal enzyme.

Taste and smell stimuli generally increase salivation. The taste sensation arises from interaction between sensors, the taste buds, on the tongue's upper surface, and dissolved constituent molecules of foods (or other ingested substances). The capability to detect four distinct sensations—sweet, sour, salt, bitter—is generally acknowledged, but the list may be longer.

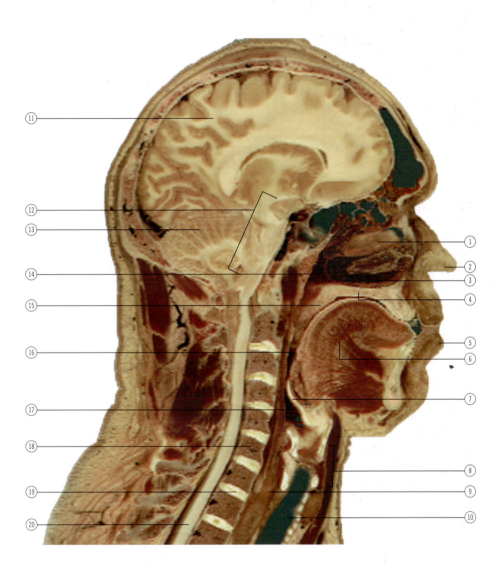

## Key

1. Nasal septum
2. External naris (nostril)
3. Nasal cavity
4. Hard palate
5. Lower lip
6. Tongue
7. Epiglottis
8. Larynx
9. Oesophagus
10. Trachea
11. Right cerebral hemisphere
12. Brainstem
13. Cerebellum
14. Nasopharynx
15. Soft palate
16. Oropharynx
17. Laryngopharynx
18. Cervical vertabra
19. Intervertebral disc
20. Spinal cord

The epiglottis, shown closed here, hinges backward slightly to open the tracheal passage. The apparent obstructions near the top of the throat are surrounding cartilages that provide structural support.

# THE OESOPHAGUS AND STOMACH

FOOD, ONCE SWALLOWED, TRAVELS DOWNWARD about a foot (25 cm) through the oesophageal tube to the stomach. The osophageal muscles work in two complementary ways to assist the descent of a food bolus, with solids taking only 4 to 8 seconds and liquids reaching the stomach even faster, in about a second.

There are two muscle layers: an inner, circular layer that constricts the **lumen**—pushing on the bolus from behind; and an outer, longitudinal layer, which pulls lengthwise—bunching or widening the lumen ahead of descending food. There is also an interior lining of friction-reducing mucous membrane. **Peristalsis**, rippling contractions of smooth muscle along the digestive tract, forces food in past the cardiac sphincter into the stomach. (The stomach's entrance is not a true sphincter, just especially well-developed muscle fibres that clinch the passage here.)

## The stomach

Shaped like a shallow, thickened crescent, the stomach is a three-layered muscle enveloping a cavity that grows or shrinks

### Key

1. Cardia (cardiac region)
2. Lesser curvature
3. Pylorus
4. Pyloric sphincter
5. Duodenum
6. Oesophagus
7. Cardiac sphincter
8. Fundus
9. Body
10. Greater curvature

The stomach's upper bulge, containing its entrance, is the fundus. Its tapered final portion is called the pylorus.

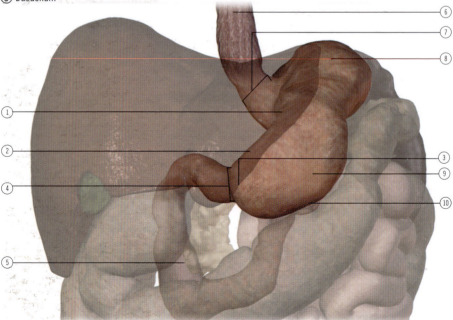

from a few ounces when empty to several quarts after a large meal. Its slight upward bulge, at the entrance, is the **fundus**; the large central mass is the body; and the lower portion, narrowing as it approaches the exit (pyloric sphincter), is the pylorus. When empty, the stomach's lining compresses itself in folds (rugae).

The stomach's muscles—arranged in outer longitudinal, middle circular, and inner oblique layers—knead and mash food. At the same time, stomach glands secrete hydrochloric acid, which degrades most foodstuffs and kills many harmful bacteria. Acid, along with mucus and **enzymes**, is produced in the stomach's lining, within millions of tiny depressions called **gastric pits**. Individual gastric glands open onto the pits' surfaces. Within the glands, parietal cells make and release the acid, about 2–3 pints (1–1.5 litres) each day. Gastric juices also contain intrinsic factor (to enable absorption of vitamin B12) and pepsin, an important enzyme that breaks down proteins into peptides, and acts most effectively in a strongly acid environment, that is, at a low pH. Were it not for a robust mucous lining, and certain secretion inhibitors called prostaglandins, the stomach could quickly erode its own internal surface and, in fact, initiate its own digestion.

Stomach secretion is activated by nerve and hormone signals. The hormone gastrin, released on eating, is the most powerful acid stimulus. Histamine, a hormone produced in the stomach lining, stimulates smooth muscle. The smell or taste of food causes an autonomic response, relayed through the vagus nerve, which may also initiate secretory activity through hormone release.

Entrance to the stomach, in the cardiac region, is not controlled by a true sphincter; the so-called cardiac sphincter does, however, narrow the access through muscular action. An unpleasant but useful consequence is that the stomach can quickly empty itself if necessary.

Cardiac opening

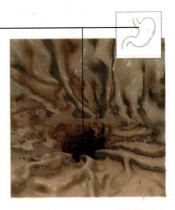

Pyloric sphincter

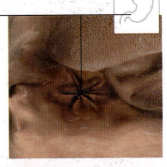

Ileocaecal opening (sphincter)

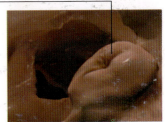

# LIVER, GALLBLADDER, AND PANCREAS

MANY OF THE ENZYMES AND SUBSTANCES needed for digestion are supplied to the small intestine by other organs, specifically by the liver and pancreas—the accessory organs to digestion. Although the liver contributes directly to digestion only by producing bile, it carries out hundreds of other operations in regulating, synthesizing, and storing nutrients. Most digestive enzymes are produced by **exocrine** cells within the pancreas. The pancreas also has a sprinkling of **endocrine** cells (the islets of Langerhans), whose function is unrelated to the digestive process.

## The liver and gallbladder

Bile, a greenish liquid, suspends fats as small droplets—i.e., it emulsifies them—so that a fat-cleaving enzyme, **lipase**, can more efficiently break them down. Bile is composed of various salts, which are mostly reabsorbed, and waste products such as cholesterol and pigment from destroyed blood cells, which pass through the digestive tract and are eliminated. On the underside of the liver, the gallbladder receives bile secreted in the liver, stores it, or expels it in response to a hormone, **cholecystokinin**, released by an active duodenum and jejunum. Bile reaches the duodenum by way of the common bile duct, which is normally joined by the pancreatic duct. The liver produces about 2 pints (one litre) of bile each day.

Beyond digestion, the liver has an exceedingly complex range of metabolic functions. Its principal cells, **hepatocytes**, assemble lipids, proteins, enzymes, clotting factors, urea, and albumin; they break down toxins, drugs, and other foreign substances; and they regulate blood glucose levels. Other kinds of liver cells repair tissue injury, store fats and vitamins (A, D, B12), or work in a similar manner to components of the immune system.

**Anterior view, showing the relationship of liver, gallbladder, pancreas, and their joint access to the duodenum, through the common bile duct.**

**Key**
① Biliary system
② Liver
③ Gallbladder
④ Major duodenal papilla
⑤ Duodenum
⑥ Oesophagus
⑦ Stomach
⑧ Common bile duct
⑨ Pancreatic duct
⑩ Pancreas

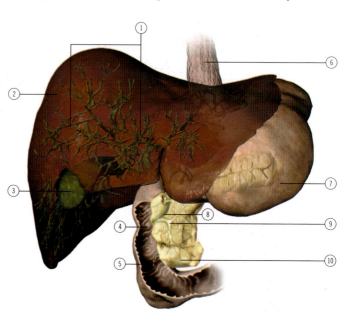

The liver is also the largest organ in the body, and its extensive metabolic activity is an important source of body heat.

Hepatocytes are stacked into plates or walls, only one cell thick, that intersect in a honeycomb arrangement; the myriad small passages between the wall segments are predominantly filled by **sinusoids**, blood channels that act like capillaries within the liver. Each small region of cells forms a cluster, called a hepatic lobule, about ¹⁄₁₆ in (1 mm) in extent, and is drained by a central vein. Sinusoids within each lobule converge to the central vein, which empties ultimately into the hepatic vein. Portal blood, venous blood entering the liver, is brought to a lobule's periphery by branching venules of the portal vein; oxygenated blood is supplied by arterial capillaries. Bile is collected differently, in a network of minute canaliculi that run between adjacent cell surfaces—that is, within the walls formed by hepatocytes.

## The pancreas

Within the pancreas, cell clusters (called **acini**) secrete digestive juices containing essential enzymes, including **amylase** (breaks down starch); **trypsin** (breaks down protein); chymotrypsinogen (an enzyme precursor); **carboxypeptidases** (take proteins apart); **lipase** (operates on fats); and **nucleases** (break down nucleic acids). A central pancreatic duct collects all tributary secretions and carries the juice to a junction with the common bile duct, and from there into the duodenum.

Pancreatic activity is stimulated by the duodenal hormones cholesystokinin and secretin, which causes secretion of sodium bicarbonate. About two pints (one litre) of digestive fluid is made in the pancreas daily. Sodium bicarbonate makes pancreatic juices strongly alkaline; together with bile, also alkaline, the mixed juices that reach the duodenum rapidly neutralize highly acidic **chyme**.

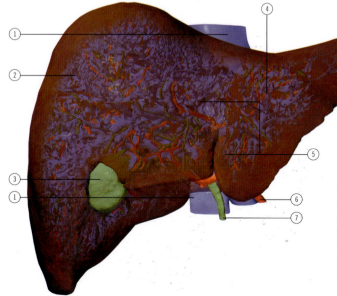

**Key**

① Inferior vena cava
② Right lobe of liver
③ Gallbladder
④ Left lobe of liver
⑤ Branches of hepatic portal vein and hepatic artery
⑥ Hepatic artery
⑦ Common bile duct

In anterior view, the liver's dense networks of arterioles and venules are seen. The gallbladder's function is to store and concentrate bile, only one of many substances produced in the liver.

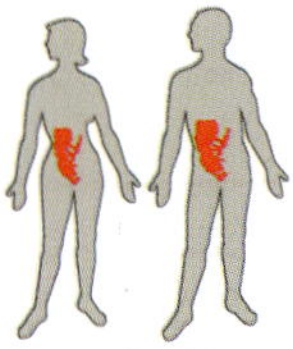

# THE SMALL INTESTINE

THE EXTRACTION OF NUTRIENTS FROM INGESTED food takes place in the small intestine, a folded tangle of smooth-muscled tubing interposed between the stomach and the large intestine. Its overall length is about 10 ft/3 m (or slightly over twice that after death, when muscle tone is absent). It contains, in order from the stomach, three segments: the duodenum (10 in/25 cm), the jejunum (3 ft/1 m), and the ileum (6 ft/2 m). Its average diameter is only about 1 in (2.5 cm).

The small intestine receives **chyme**— food that has been churned by the stomach to a pasty consistency—and mixes it with bile, pancreatic juices, and enzymes to break it down into usable nutrient forms, which are absorbed through the intestinal walls.

First, however, the highly acidic chyme must be neutralized; this is accomplished in the duodenum with sodium bicarbonate, which is produced in the pancreas. Ducts bringing digestive juices from both the liver and pancreas converge at the duodenum.

Longitudinal and circular layers of smooth muscle generate a rhythmic peristaltic push. In the small intestine, however, waves of circular contractions alone also occur, a squeezing action termed **segmentation** that further mixes food and digestive juices. Along the inner wall, particularly in the jejunum, encircling ridges line the intestinal **lumen**. Called **plicae circulares**, these

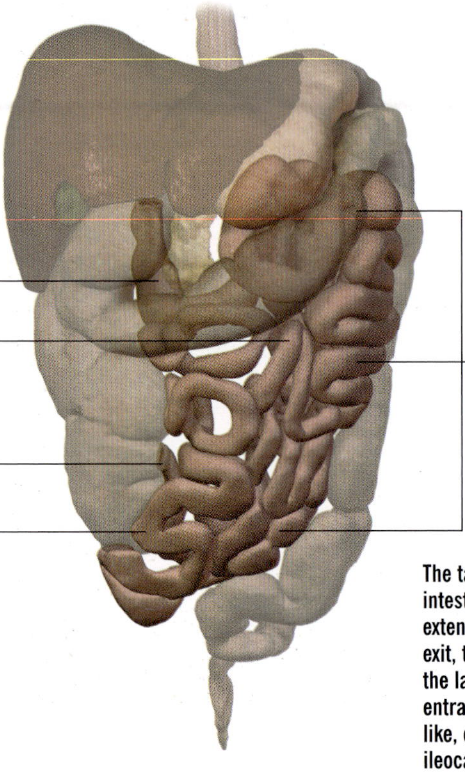

Duodenum

Jejunum

Junction with the large intestine

Ileum

Small intestine

**The tangle of the small intestine, in anterior view, extends from the stomach's exit, the pyloric sphincter, to the large intestine's entrance, at the sphincter-like, double-flapped ileocaecal valve.**

are folds of mucous membrane about ½ in (10 mm) high. The plicae and the spaces between them are covered in **villi**, fingerlike projections 1/16 in (1 mm) long. The folds and carpet of villi compact a great deal of surface into the intestine's length, increasing its effective contact area by a factor of several hundred times compared to a bare-walled tube. The plicae, in turn, are densely covered in microvilli (about 200 million in every 1/20 in squared/per square millimeter), to which are attached certain digestive enzymes. These are, however, only the final components in a thorough enzymatic processing, one that begins in the mouth, with the salivary enzymes, and also involves a large group of pancreatic enzymes.

The villus is really the working unit of digestion. Within each villus are found blood capillaries and a lymphatic vessel called a **lacteal**. Enzymes carried on the microvilli—which are termed **brush border enzymes**—cleave sugars and peptides (the subparts of most proteins) into simpler substances. The enzymes **maltase**, **sucrase**, and **lactase** reduce complex sugars to simple ones (such as glucose or fructose); other enzymes, **peptidases**, break peptide bonds between amino acids.

Simple sugars and amino acids enter the circulation through capillaries within the villus. Fatty acids and glycerol recombine as fats inside the villus and are taken up in the lacteals, for eventual transport into the bloodstream.

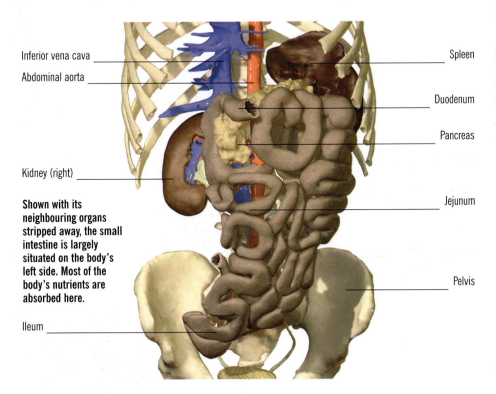

Inferior vena cava

Abdominal aorta

Kidney (right)

**Shown with its neighbouring organs stripped away, the small intestine is largely situated on the body's left side. Most of the body's nutrients are absorbed here.**

Ileum

Spleen

Duodenum

Pancreas

Jejunum

Pelvis

# THE LARGE INTESTINE

EVERYTHING THAT IS NOT EXTRACTED OR absorbed in the small intestine will be processed as waste in the large intestine, the end of the line for ingested material. About 3 pints (1.5 litres) of watery material enters the large intestine every day and is reduced to a somewhat more solid 8–12 oz (200–300 g) of residue. A population of trillions of bacteria transforms undigested substances into a semisolid mass called feces—accomplished during a slow progress along the large intestine's 5-foot (1.5-m) length. The bacteria, quite harmful if not isolated from other body systems (or from food and water supplies), make up 25 percent or more of the solid content of material ultimately expelled.

The large intestine consists of four segments: the caecum, colon, rectum, and anal canal; separation from the small intestine is marked by the ileocaecal valve, entering from the ilium, which prevents reflux of intestinal contents once past this point. Its diameter, 3 in (6.5 cm), is about twice that of the small intestine. The colon takes a long path—first up, across, down, and then in an S-shaped section at the end—to the terminal segments, the rectum and anal canal. Sections are named, accordingly, by their direction: the ascending, transverse, descending, and sigmoid colon. Passage through the rectum is controlled by two rings of muscle, which are termed the internal and external sphincters.

As in most of the organs along the digestive tube, the muscles making up the colon's outer coat are in two layers: inner circumferential fibres, and outer longitudinal muscle. In this case, the longitudinal fibres are gathered together in three bands called **teniae coli**

("ribbons of the colon"). The long fibres tend to shorten segments of the colon, creating pouchy bulges called **haustra** along its length. Their numbers and appearance fluctuate according to the activity of the colon.

Undigested matter passes into the caecum in a semi-liquid state. Along the large intestine's internal lining, water is absorbed into blood capillaries; this is an important means of maintaining the body's fluid balance. The gradually solidifying contents are forwarded by **peristalsis**. The time of transit is normally about 10 to 12 hours; movement is steady and unrestricted. When the stomach receives food, peristaltic action intensifies for a while, pushing everything along more quickly.

The need to defecate—to expel fecal material—arises when an already full sigmoid colon propels feces into the rectum. The rectal walls stretch, causing awareness of its content. Defecation can then take place if its sphincters are consciously relaxed, thus opening an exit through the short anal canal. Folds inside the rectum, where it bends sharply in three places, aid in separating **flatus** (bacterially produced gas) from feces. The folds, called **rectal valves**, impede solid passage, while gas may reach the anus and be expelled separately.

## The appendix

Attached to the caecum's back side, just as it joins the ascending colon, is the appendix, a narrow closed tube, about 4 in (9 cm) long. Though it has a digestive function in some animals, it has long been thought nonfunctional in human beings. It is rich in lymphatic tissue, however, and research suggests the appendix may have a role in immune system defences.

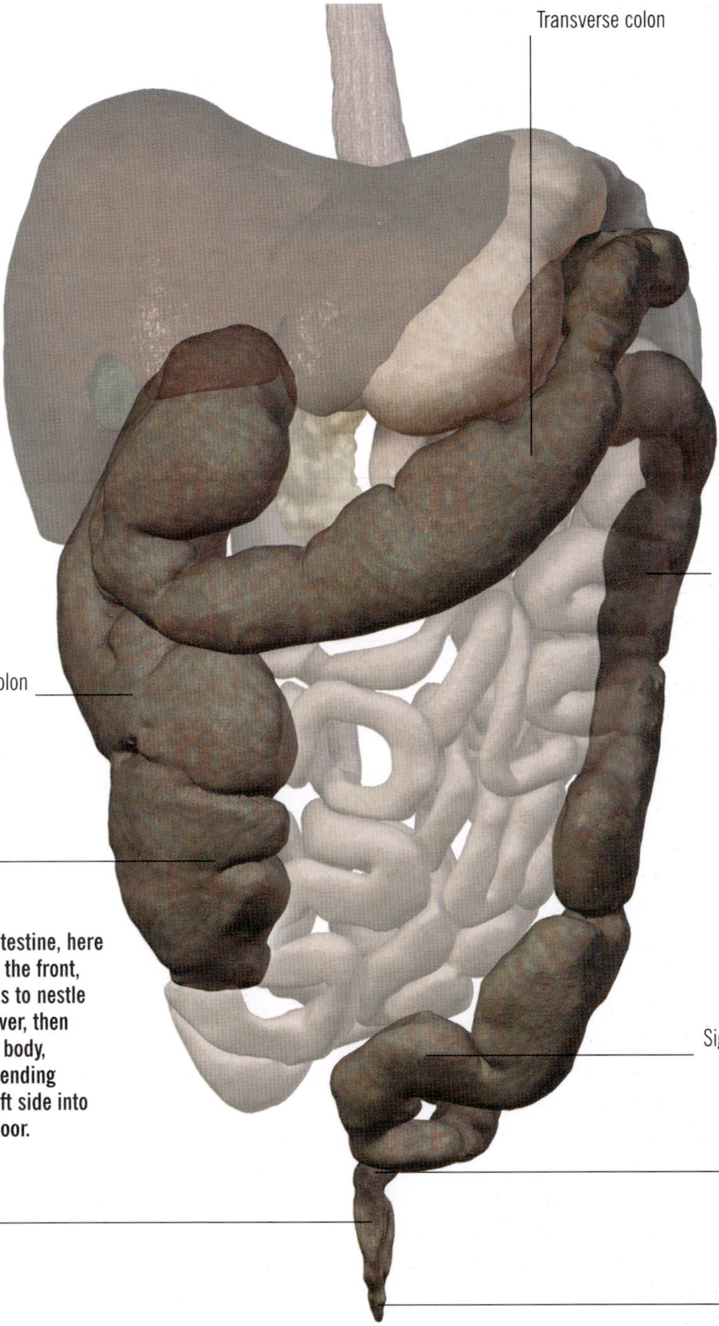

Transverse colon

Descending
colon

Ascending colon

Caecum

The large intestine, here
shown from the front,
first ascends to nestle
under the liver, then
crosses the body,
before descending
along the left side into
the pelvic floor.

Sigmoid colon

Rectum

Anal canal

Anus

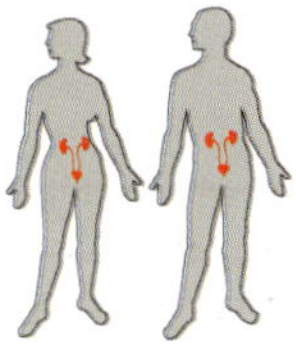

# THE URINARY SYSTEM

THE URINARY SYSTEM CLEANSES THE BLOOD of waste materials and maintains its proper concentration of sodium chloride and other substances. The most important organs in the system are the two kidneys, whose waste-processing activities result in the production of **urine**, which is stored in the bladder and excreted via the urethra.

About 5 in (12 cm) long and 3 in (6 cm) wide, the kidneys are located in the upper abdominal cavity, one on either side of the backbone. Each is protected and supported by three layers of tissue. The outer layer, the **renal fascia**, holds the kidney against the abdominal wall.

A front view of the abdominal area showing the location of the kidneys, ureters, bladder, and urethra. In males, as shown here, the urethra passes through the penis. In females, it opens in the vulva.

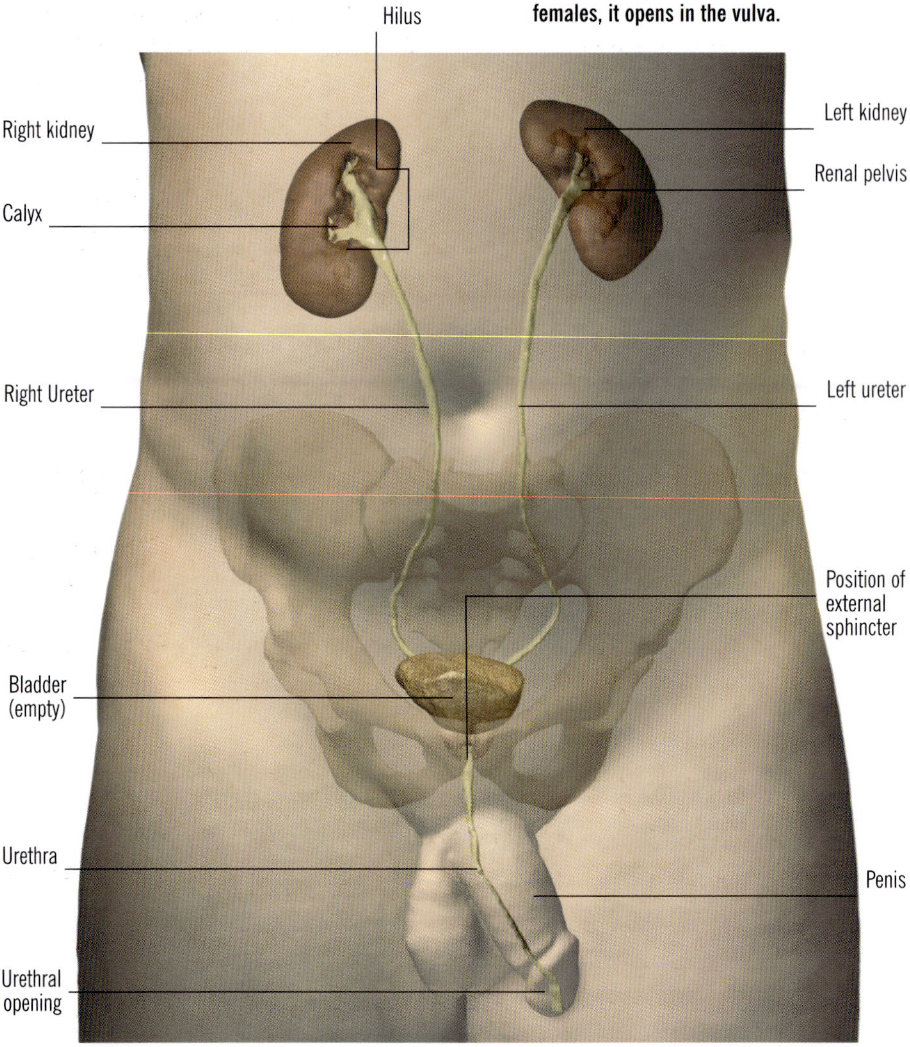

Hilus

Right kidney

Calyx

Left kidney

Renal pelvis

Right Ureter

Left ureter

Position of external sphincter

Bladder (empty)

Urethra

Penis

Urethral opening

The inner layer, the **renal capsule**, helps insulate it from infection. In the middle is a cushioning layer of **adipose** (fat) tissue.

The kidneys filter from the blood dissolved waste produced by metabolic activity, drugs, and other toxins. They also maintain the proper balance of fluid, salts, and acid in the body by adjusting the amounts retained and excreted. About ¼ teaspoon (1 ml) of urine is produced a minute. It is transported into the bladder for storage through the ureters, long muscular tubes (16–18 in/40–45 cm) that press urine onward in **peristaltic** waves.

The bladder is a muscular bag connecting to the urethra at the internal urethral sphincter. This ring of muscle, which is not under conscious control, holds the urine within the bladder.

Below it, the pelvic floor muscles form the external urethral sphincter, which operates voluntarily. When the bladder contains between 10 and 14 oz (300–400 ml) of urine, the wall is sufficiently stretched that sensory receptors send nerve impulses to the spinal cord; the impulses cause the internal sphincter to open and create a feeling of the need to urinate. When the external sphincter is voluntarily relaxed, the bladder wall muscles contract and urine is forced out through the urethra.

A view of the kidneys showing the adrenal glands that sit atop them, and the renal veins and arteries that carry blood to and from the kidneys for filtration.

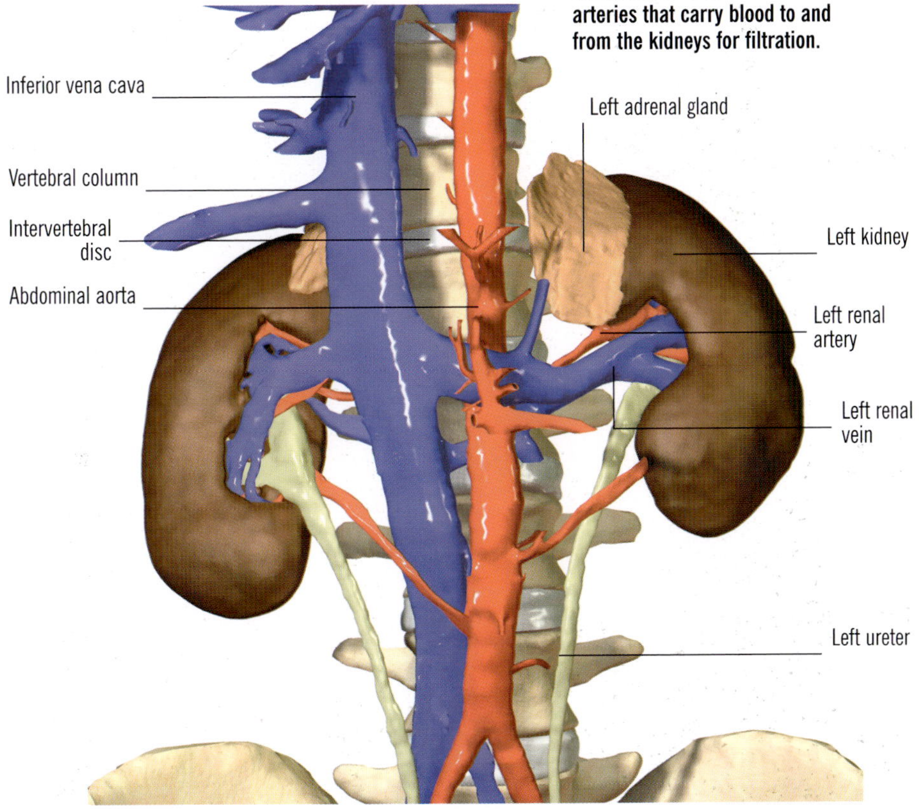

Inferior vena cava

Vertebral column

Intervertebral disc

Abdominal aorta

Left adrenal gland

Left kidney

Left renal artery

Left renal vein

Left ureter

# THE KIDNEYS

THE KIDNEYS FILTER
THE ENTIRE BLOOD
supply about 20 times per
hour. Filtering is accomplished by
approximately one million microscopic
tubes in each kidney called **nephrons**.
These remove small molecules and ions
from the blood, reclaim materials needed
by the body, and leave the surplus and
waste to flow out as urine.

Each kidney consists of an outer
cortex and inner medulla, and the renal
pelvis, a hollow funnel connecting the
kidney to the ureter. The inner surface of
the medulla is formed of **medullary
pyramids**. Looping between the cortex
and medulla are the nephrons. Each has a
**renal tubule**, closed at one end and
open at the other, and a network of

**Key**

① Inferior vena cava
② Common hepatic
   artery
③ Splenic artery
④ Coeliac trunk
⑤ Superior
   mesenteric artery
⑥ Thoracic vertebra
⑦ Intervertebral disc
⑧ Abdominal aorta
⑨ Branches of renal
   artery and vein
   inside kidney
⑩ Left renal artery
⑪ Left kidney
⑫ Left renal vein
⑬ Left ureter

A frontal view of the left
kidney in the upper
abdomen, showing the
renal vein and artery
entering through the
hilus. The lowest ribs,
branching off the upper
lumbar section of the
spine, offer the kidneys
some protection.

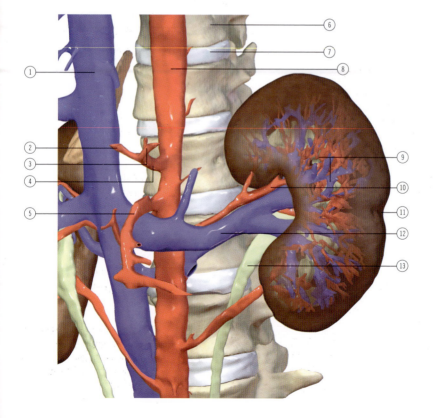

capillaries called the **glomerulus**. Pressure inside the glomerulus causes liquid from the blood to flow into the glomerular capsule, located at the closed end of the tubule. Both waste products and useful substances pass into the tubule. As the liquid passes along the looped tubule, waste products are retained, while glucose and amino acids, most of the liquid, and salts are resorbed (reabsorbed) into the blood.

A major waste component is **urea**, which is a nitrogen–containing (**nitrogenous**) compound formed when the liver combines carbon dioxide with ammonia, a highly poisonous byproduct of excess amino acids.

The amount of salts and water resorbed is regulated by the hormones, so that bodily concentrations are maintained at optimal levels. Urine is composed of the remaining fluid and waste after resorption. It passes into the renal pelvis through the **calyces**, cup-shaped branches of collecting ducts that cover the tops of the medullary pyramids.

Although the kidneys represent only about 0.5 percent of body weight, they receive directly up to 25 percent of the blood pumped by the heart. Blood vessels, as well as lymph vessels and nerves, enter and exit the kidney at an indentation, or hilus, that leads to a space called the **renal sinus**. The renal artery, a branch of the aorta, carries blood into the kidney. The artery branches into a number of smaller arteries that pass between the medullary pyramids and into the cortex.

Venous branches in the cortex join into the renal vein, which carries blood from the kidney and drains ultimately into the inferior vena cava.

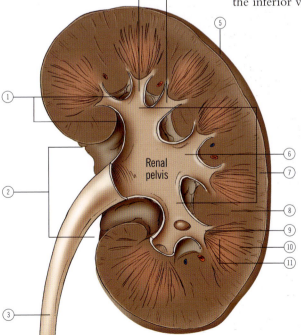

Renal pelvis

**Key**
1. Renal sinus
2. Hilus
3. Ureter
4. Minor calyces
5. Fibrous capsule
6. Major calyces
7. Cortex
8. Renal column
9. Papilla of pyramid
10. Base of pyramid
11. Medulla (pyramid)

**A cross-sectional diagram of the left kidney. The microscopic nephrons loop between the medulla and cortex and empty into the calyces.**

# THE MALE REPRODUCTIVE SYSTEM

THE REPRODUCTIVE SYSTEM TAKES DIFFERENT FORMS in males and females, and contributions from each are required for the creation of offspring. In both sexes the system matures at **puberty**, at which time the body also takes on male or female secondary sexual characteristics. Sex cells are produced in the male testes and female ovaries. Fertilization of a female sex cell (egg) by a male sex cell (sperm) leads to the development of a fetus inside the female uterus.

Initially, the external genitalia of male and female embryos are identical. In males, the Y chromosome initiates the development of testes. The testes begin to secrete **testosterone**, which causes the previously undifferentiated external genitalia to grow into a penis and scrotum. In the absence of a Y chromosome, female external genitalia, the clitoris and labia, are formed from the same tissue.

The male reproductive system consists of the two testes, the penis, the ducts that connect testes to penis, and the accessory glands, i.e., the seminal vesicle and prostate gland. The primary male sex organs are the testes, where sperm is produced. The two testes are suspended outside and below the pelvic cavity inside a sac called the scrotum. The location of the scrotum outside the body allows the temperature in the testes to remain some 5 degrees F (3 degrees C) below core body temperature, which is optimal for sperm production.

Millions of sperm are produced every day; each consists of a head containing genetic material and a tail, or **flagellum**, which propels the sperm through bodily fluids. Sperm are produced in the walls of compartments in the coiled seminiferous tubules by the division of sperm-making germ cells. Immature sperm pass along the seminiferous tubules to the epididymis, a coiled structure running along the back of the testis, where they mature over two or three weeks.

Sperm production is controlled by the pituitary hormones **luteinizing hormone** (LH) and **follicle-stimulating hormone** (FSH). LH stimulates the release of testosterone from the interstitial cells that surround the seminiferous tubules; testosterone stimulates the tubules to produce sperm. FSH aids in sperm production by concentrating testosterone around the sperm-producing cells.

**Key**

1. Iliac bone of pelvis
2. Bladder
3. Prostatic urethra
4. Prostate gland
5. Membranous urethra
6. Epididymis
7. Scrotum
8. Testis
9. Sacrum
10. Kidney
11. Testicular artery and vein
12. Ureter
13. Pelvis
14. Ductus deferens
15. Pubic bone of pelvis
16. Crus of penis
17. Corpus cavernosum
18. Penile urethra
19. Glans penis

The male reproductive organs are the testes, the penis, the ducts that connect the testes to the penis, and the accessory glands (the seminal vesicle and prostate gland). Sperm are produced in the testes and carried to the penis via the vas deferens, while the seminal vesicle and prostate gland release secretions that form semen. The penis, which transfers sperm out of the body, also forms part of the urinary system.

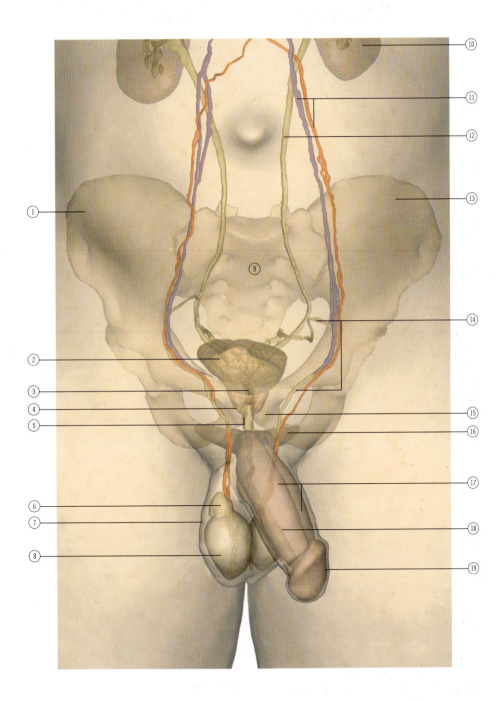

# THE MALE REPRODUCTIVE SYSTEM

THE PENIS IS THE ORGAN THAT enables the transfer of sperm into the female vagina during sexual intercourse. It is cylindrical in shape, and is composed of the root, which attaches to the pubic arch, the body or shaft, and an expanded tip, the glans. Inside the shaft is the corpus spongiosum, which surrounds the urethra, the duct that carries both semen and urine out of the body. The corpus spongiosum, along with two corpora cavernosa that run along the sides of the upper part of the shaft, enlarge when engorged with blood during an erection.

A cross-sectional view of the male reproductive system showing the path by which sperm are transferred from the testes through the vas deferens to the urethra, as well as the accessory glands that secrete the components of semen.

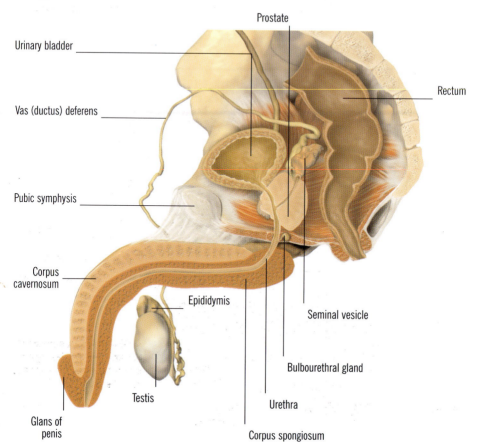

Prostate

Urinary bladder

Rectum

Vas (ductus) deferens

Pubic symphysis

Corpus cavernosum

Epididymis

Seminal vesicle

Bulbourethral gland

Glans of penis

Testis

Urethra

Corpus spongiosum

# Release of sperm

For sperm to be released from the penis into the female vagina, erection and ejaculation must occur. These processes are controlled by two reflexes triggered by the autonomic nervous system (ANS). First, during sexual arousal, the ANS reflexively causes the blood vessels in the penis to widen, increasing blood flow to the organ. This increase causes the spongy tissues of the corpus spongiosum and corpora cavernosa to expand. The penis becomes enlarged and stiff.

As sexual arousal reaches its peak, the ANS sets off a two-stage ejaculation reflex. In the first stage, the two vasa deferentia (plural of vas deferens) contract and press sperm through the urethra to the base of the penis, while the seminal vesicle and prostate (accessory glands) release secretions into the vasa and urethra, which combine to form the semen that carries, activates, and energizes the sperm. Following this first phase, muscles at the base of the penis contract up to 5 times at 0.8 second intervals, propelling the sperm-carrying semen out through the urethra. Approximately one teaspoon (5 ml) of semen is released, holding an average of 300 million sperm. After ejaculation, the erection ceases.

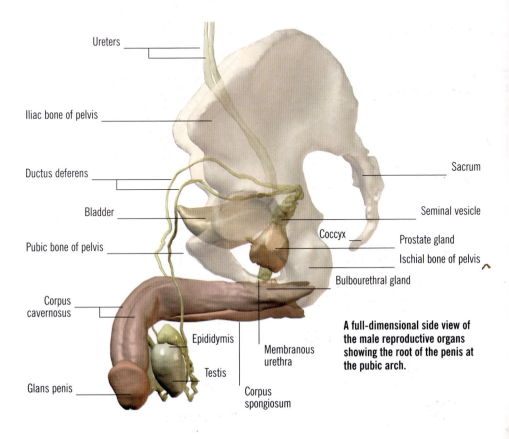

Ureters

Iliac bone of pelvis

Ductus deferens

Bladder

Pubic bone of pelvis

Corpus cavernosus

Glans penis

Epididymis

Testis

Membranous urethra

Corpus spongiosum

Sacrum

Seminal vesicle

Coccyx

Prostate gland

Ischial bone of pelvis

Bulbourethral gland

**A full-dimensional side view of the male reproductive organs showing the root of the penis at the pubic arch.**

# THE FEMALE REPRODUCTIVE SYSTEM

THE FEMALE REPRODUCTIVE SYSTEM CONTAINS THE eggs, or ova, which are the female sex cells, and, in pregnancy, the developing fetus. It consists of the ovaries, where eggs mature; the uterus, where the fetus grows and develops; the Fallopian tubes, through which the eggs travel from the ovaries to the uterus; the cervix, or neck of the uterus; the vagina, which opens to the exterior of the body; and the external genitals, the labia and clitoris.

## The ovaries and the ovarian cycle

The paired ovaries are located on either side of the uterus near the ends of the uterine (Fallopian) tubes. These not only house the female sex cells, they also secrete the female sex hormones oestrogen and progesterone. The ovaries contain up to 2 million immature eggs at birth, encased in follicles, or sacs. No new eggs are produced during a woman's lifetime.

Each month, the pituitary hormone **follicle-stimulating hormone** (FSH) stimulates some of the follicles to grow. Influenced by a surge of **luteinizing hormone** (LH), another pituitary hormone, ovulation occurs: one egg enlarges to maturity, bursts out of its follicle, and is released into the Fallopian tube. The mature ovum has only half the number of chromosomes it originally contained. Following ovulation the remains of the follicle become the corpus luteum, which produces oestrogen and progesterone. If no pregnancy occurs, the corpus luteum begins to degenerate, and hormonal production declines, initiating the next ovarian cycle.

## The menstrual cycle

Ovulation occurs two weeks into the approximately 28-day female reproductive cycle. By this time, stimulated by increased oestrogen levels, the endometrium (the lining of the uterus) has begun to thicken. Following ovulation, and under the influence of the hormone progesterone, it thickens further, preparing to support a pregnancy. If no pregnancy occurs, hormonal production declines quickly and a period occurs.

**Key (top)**
1. Iliac bone of pelvis
2. Sacrum
3. Pubic bone of pelvis
4. Ischial bone of pelvis
5. Infundibulum of uterine tube
6. Ovary
7. Uterine tube
8. Uterus
9. Bladder
10. Vagina

**Key (bottom)**
1. Sacrum
2. Iliac crest
3. Ilium
4. Vagina
5. Infundibulum of uterine tube
6. Uterine tube
7. Pubis
8. Bladder
9. Uterus
10. External iliac vein
11. External iliac artery
12. Ovarian artery and vein
13. Uterine arteries and veins
14. Ovary

Front view of the female pelvis (*above*) showing the location of the main female reproductive organs.

Superior view of the female pelvic cavity (*below*) showing the reproductive organs in relation to other structures, with associated veins and arteries.

# THE FEMALE REPRODUCTIVE SYSTEM

ALTHOUGH THE OVARIES ARE CONSIDERED TO BE the primary female sexual organ, other elements of the reproductive system are involved in sexual intercourse, egg fertilization, fetal development, and, finally, childbirth.

• The Fallopian tubes are narrow ducts about 4 in (10 cm) long that run from the ovaries to the uterus. Fertilization occurs within one of the tubes, which carries the fertilized egg into the uterus, where the egg is implanted and fetal development begins.

• The uterus is a hollow muscular organ located in front of the rectum and behind the bladder and held in place by ligaments. Its outer layer is the perimetrium, within which is a thick layer of smooth muscle, the myometrium. The endometrium, a layer of soft tissue that lines the uterus, is the site at which the fertilized egg is implanted. The myometrium of the uterus expands greatly during pregnancy. At the end of pregnancy, it is the powerful rhythmic contractions of the myometrium that initiate childbirth.

**A cross-section of the female pelvis showing the internal and external reproductive organs, from the ovary at the top to the labia minora at the bottom.**

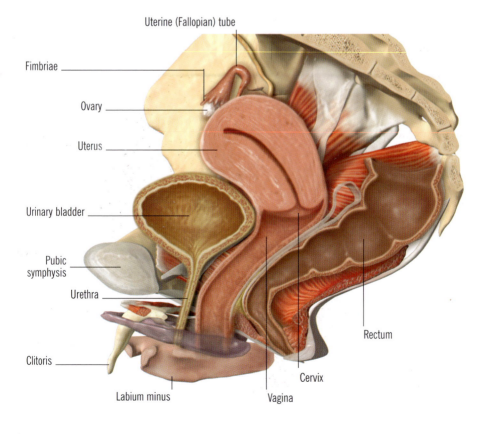

Uterine (Fallopian) tube

Fimbriae

Ovary

Uterus

Urinary bladder

Pubic symphysis

Urethra

Clitoris

Labium minus

Vagina

Cervix

Rectum

- The cervix is the neck of the uterus, by which it connects to the vagina. During pregnancy, the opening of the cervix remains small, but in later stages its connective tissues soften, permitting passage of the fetus from the uterus into the vagina.
- The vagina is a muscular tube 3–4 in (8–10 cm) in length that connects the uterus to the outside of the body. During intercourse, the penis is inserted into it, permitting ejaculated sperm to move into the uterus and Fallopian tubes. Endometrial tissues pass out through it during menstruation, and in childbirth it expands to permit the baby to exit the body.

- The external genitalia, or vulva, is made up of the labia and clitoris. The labia majora and minora protect the vaginal and urethral openings, and the clitoris. The clitoris is the female homologue of the penis and is the main site of sexual arousal. In common with the penis, it consists of a glans and shaft, and contains erectile tissue. Although it is a much smaller structure than the penis, it also contains an intricate network of blood vessels and neurons.

**A side view of the female pelvis showing the internal reproductive organs and their relationship to the bones of the pelvis and sacrum.**

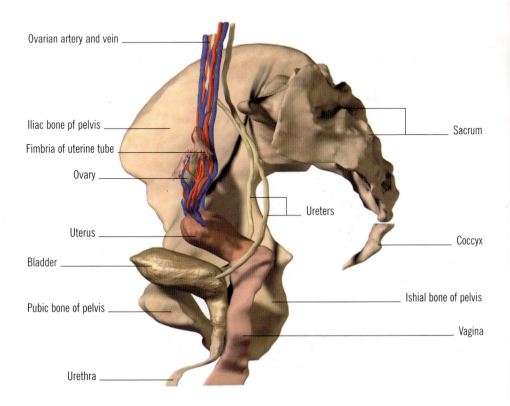

Ovarian artery and vein

Iliac bone pf pelvis

Fimbria of uterine tube

Ovary

Uterus

Bladder

Pubic bone of pelvis

Urethra

Sacrum

Ureters

Coccyx

Ishial bone of pelvis

Vagina

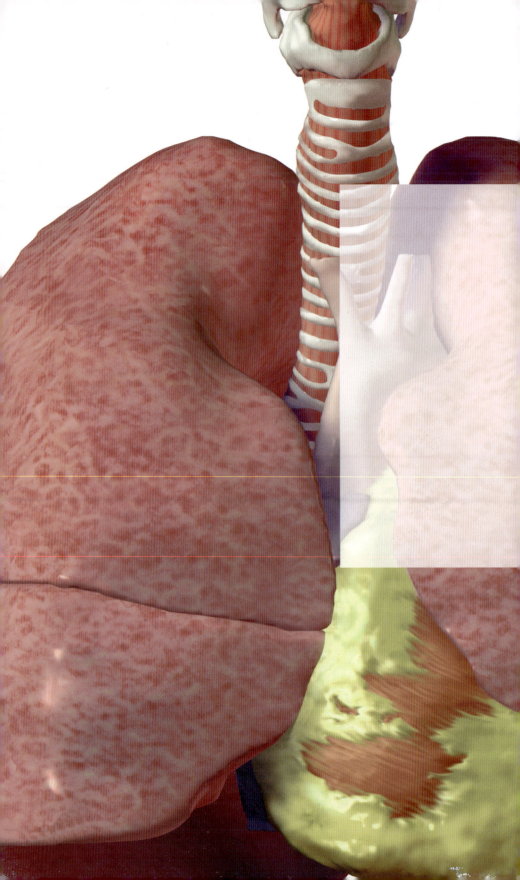

# REGIONAL ANATOMY

A regional approach to anatomy looks at body tissues in isolation, and is most useful for conveying a sense of the way the body actually looks, rather than describing how different parts of the body work together within a whole system.

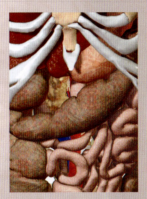

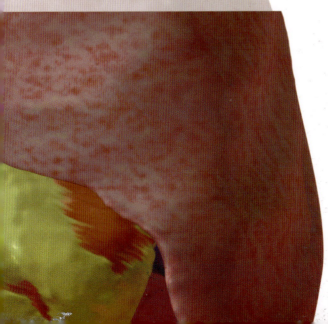

# THE HEAD AND NECK

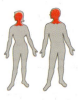

THE PROTECTIVE SKULL HOUSES THE BRAIN and sensory organs, as well as containing the openings through which we take in nourishment and air. Supported by the seven **cervical vertebrae**, the neck links the head to the body, holds it in position, and provides it with a range of motion.

## The muscles

The muscles of the head and neck are largely controlled by the cranial nerves. Superficial scalp muscles, such as the frontalis, and face muscles, such as the zygomaticus, produce facial expressions by pulling on the skin. There are more than 30 small facial muscles altogether.

The jaw is controlled by four mastication (chewing) muscles, including the temporalis, which pull the jaw upward, and smaller muscles that move it from side to side. Muscles at the front of the neck are used for swallowing, while those at the back extend and support the head. The sternocleidomastoid muscles flex and tilt the head. Within the mouth, the tongue muscles protract and retract it and move it from side to side.

### Key

① Temporalis
② Levator labii superioris alaeque nasi
③ Nasal cartilage
④ External jugular vein
⑤ Facial vein
⑥ Mentalis
⑦ External carotid artery
⑧ Sternocleidomastoid
⑨ Frontalis
⑩ Orbicularis oculi
⑪ Levator labii superioris
⑫ Zygomaticus minor
⑬ Zygomaticus major
⑭ Orbicularis oris
⑮ Depressor anguli oris
⑯ Depressor labii inferioris
⑰ Sternohyoid
⑱ Larynx

Front view of the head and neck showing the superficial muscles. The muscles of the face are unusual because they insert directly into the skin.

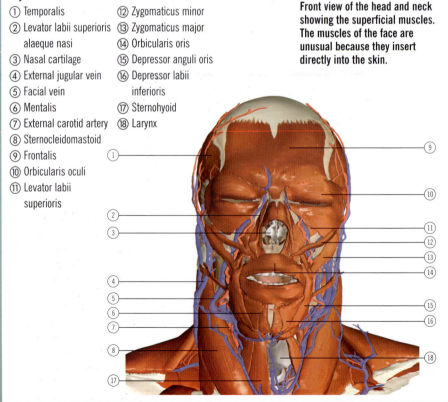

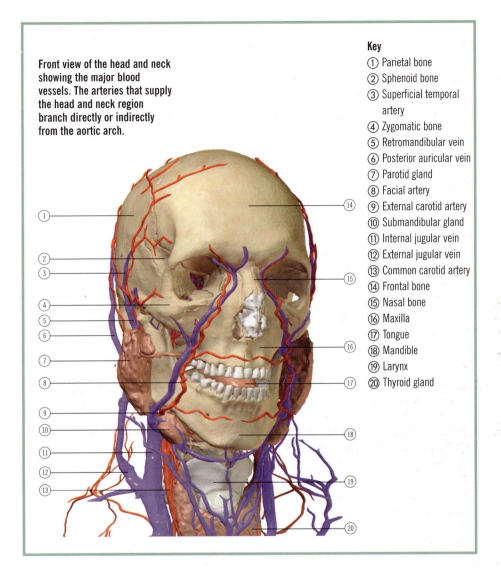

Front view of the head and neck showing the major blood vessels. The arteries that supply the head and neck region branch directly or indirectly from the aortic arch.

**Key**
1. Parietal bone
2. Sphenoid bone
3. Superficial temporal artery
4. Zygomatic bone
5. Retromandibular vein
6. Posterior auricular vein
7. Parotid gland
8. Facial artery
9. External carotid artery
10. Submandibular gland
11. Internal jugular vein
12. External jugular vein
13. Common carotid artery
14. Frontal bone
15. Nasal bone
16. Maxilla
17. Tongue
18. Mandible
19. Larynx
20. Thyroid gland

# Blood supply

Most tissues of the head and neck are supplied with blood by the carotid arteries. Each divides into an external and internal branch; the external branch serves the head, while the internal branch supplies most of the brain and the eye region. The cerebellum and part of the cerebrum, as well as the neck, are served by the vertebral arteries. Blood drains from the head through the jugular veins, which, like the carotid arteries, divide into an internal branch that serves the brain and an external branch that serves the rest of the head. The vertebral veins drain blood from the neck.

# The tongue

The tongue is primarily composed of muscle. Its surface is covered with three types of protrusions called papillae: filiform papillae make the surface uneven, thereby helping the tongue to hold onto food. The fungiform and circumvallate papillae contain the taste buds.

# THE BRAIN

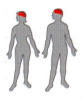

THE BRAIN IS ENCASED WITHIN THE dome-shaped cranial bones. The skull and facial bones protect the eyes and other specialized sensory organs that communicate directly with the brain. Attached to the back of the brain, and continuous with the brainstem, is the spinal cord.

## Internal structures

The lowest part of the brain is the brainstem, which consists, in ascending order, of the medulla oblongata, the pons, and the midbrain. These regions control unconscious functions, such as the heart and breathing rates, as well as unconscious muscular activity.

Above the brainstem are the thalamus, a very important relay station for sensory information, and the hypothalamus, which has interconnections with various parts of

the limbic system and outputs that influence the pituitary gland.

Close to the inner border of each cerebral hemisphere is a horseshoe-shaped area called the limbic lobe, which houses components of the limbic system, or emotional brain. The hippocampus and amygdala are important parts of the limbic system, as well as having an important role in memory. The fornix is a link among components of the system.

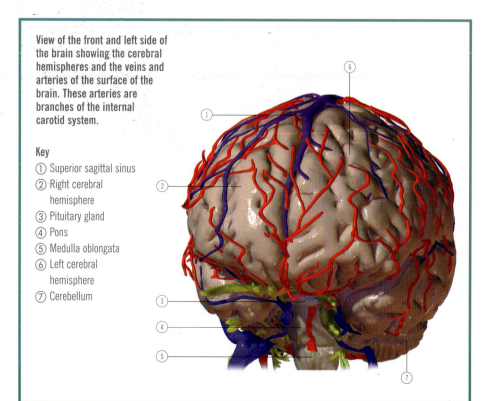

View of the front and left side of the brain showing the cerebral hemispheres and the veins and arteries of the surface of the brain. These arteries are branches of the internal carotid system.

Key
1. Superior sagittal sinus
2. Right cerebral hemisphere
3. Pituitary gland
4. Pons
5. Medulla oblongata
6. Left cerebral hemisphere
7. Cerebellum

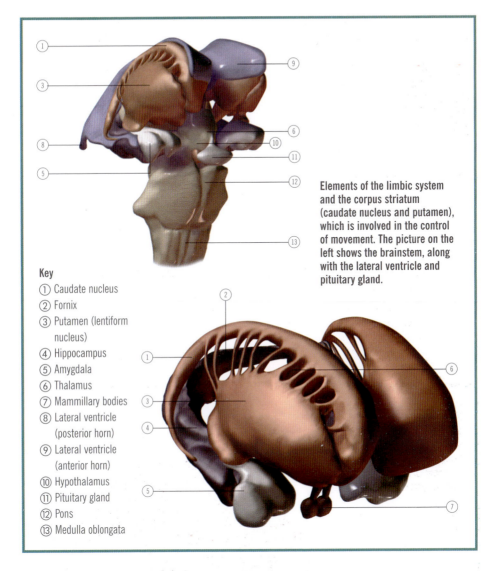

Elements of the limbic system and the corpus striatum (caudate nucleus and putamen), which is involved in the control of movement. The picture on the left shows the brainstem, along with the lateral ventricle and pituitary gland.

**Key**
1. Caudate nucleus
2. Fornix
3. Putamen (lentiform nucleus)
4. Hippocampus
5. Amygdala
6. Thalamus
7. Mammillary bodies
8. Lateral ventricle (posterior horn)
9. Lateral ventricle (anterior horn)
10. Hypothalamus
11. Pituitary gland
12. Pons
13. Medulla oblongata

## Protection of the brain

The brain is suspended within a series of three membranous coverings called **meninges**: the outer dura mater, the arachnoid mater, and the inner pia mater. These stabilize the position of the brain in two ways. First, the meninges are anchored to the skull, so that the brain must move along with the head. Second, beneath the arachnoid mater is a layer of **cerebrospinal** fluid that, by surrounding the brain, cushions it against bumps and jolts. The protective layers around the brain also serve to control the brain's environment by insulating it to some extent from the rest of the body.

# THE THORAX

THE TRUNK DIVIDES INTO TWO LARGE regions, the thorax and abdomen. The thorax is the upper segment—from the neck to abdomen—housing the lungs and heart within an area enclosed by the sternum, vertebral column, encircling ribs and costal cartilages, and associated major muscles.

Collectively, organs within the trunk are referred to as the viscera.

In the thorax, each lung is surrounded by a single pleural cavity, or space. Each cavity is lined by a sheet of cells, or **pleura**, which produces a thin layer of fluid that fills the narrow pleural space between the lung and the chest wall. The pleura applied to the lungs is known as visceral pleura, and the pleura coating the chest wall is called parietal pleura. Because pleural fluid cannot expand, the lungs remain closely applied to the chest wall during breathing movements.

The diaphragm muscle, which originates in the lower border of the ribcage and sternum, the lower costal cartilages, and the lumbar vertebrae, forms the boundary between the thoracic and the abdominopelvic cavity. It plays the chief part in respiration. When relaxed, the diaphragm is dome-shaped, but on contraction it flattens, pushing the abdominal contents downward, expanding the thorax, and drawing air into the lungs. On relaxing, it becomes dome-shaped once again, and pushes air out of the lungs.

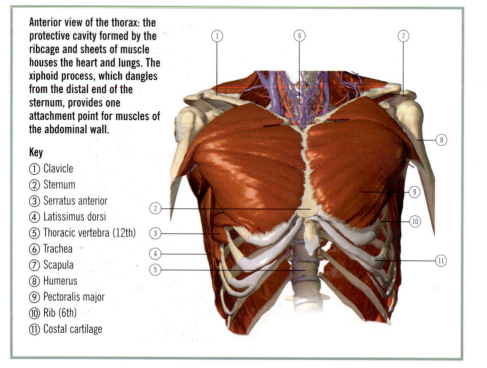

Anterior view of the thorax: the protective cavity formed by the ribcage and sheets of muscle houses the heart and lungs. The xiphoid process, which dangles from the distal end of the sternum, provides one attachment point for muscles of the abdominal wall.

**Key**
1. Clavicle
2. Sternum
3. Serratus anterior
4. Latissimus dorsi
5. Thoracic vertebra (12th)
6. Trachea
7. Scapula
8. Humerus
9. Pectoralis major
10. Rib (6th)
11. Costal cartilage

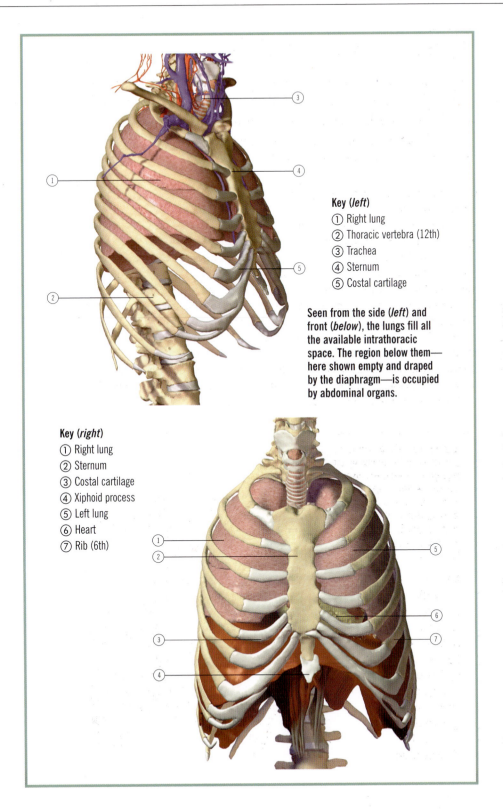

**Key (*left*)**
① Right lung
② Thoracic vertebra (12th)
③ Trachea
④ Sternum
⑤ Costal cartilage

Seen from the side (*left*) and front (*below*), the lungs fill all the available intrathoracic space. The region below them— here shown empty and draped by the diaphragm—is occupied by abdominal organs.

**Key (*right*)**
① Right lung
② Sternum
③ Costal cartilage
④ Xiphoid process
⑤ Left lung
⑥ Heart
⑦ Rib (6th)

# THE THORAX

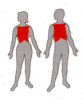

BETWEEN THE TWO PLEURAE AND EXTENDING from the spinal column forward to the sternum is an internal space called the **mediastinum**. Within this corridor between the lungs are located the heart, its trunk arteries and veins, and the oesophagus and trachea.

The heart's fitted mediastinal space, almost surrounded by the lungs, is called the cardiac impression. The parietal pleura defining the space joins at its base with the visceral pleurae of the lungs, sealing the pleural space. Descending into the abdominal cavity, the oesophagus, aorta, and inferior vena cava pierce the diaphragm into three openings, which are called foramina.

A pulmonary ligament ties the lungs firmly to the diaphragm, holding them in place and expanding them downward during inspiration. The diaphragm, controlled by the phrenic nerve, is the chief muscle of breathing, assisted by the intercostal muscles—especially in forced expiration—which spread the ribs or pull them together.

## The superficial muscles

The superficial thoracic muscles are in the form of flat, overlying sheets, which are tied together at the front and back by seams of connective fascia. Their outermost layer includes the pectoralis

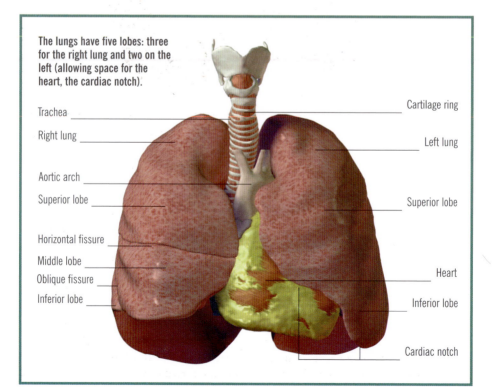

The lungs have five lobes: three for the right lung and two on the left (allowing space for the heart, the cardiac notch).

Trachea

Right lung

Aortic arch

Superior lobe

Horizontal fissure

Middle lobe

Oblique fissure

Inferior lobe

Cartilage ring

Left lung

Superior lobe

Heart

Inferior lobe

Cardiac notch

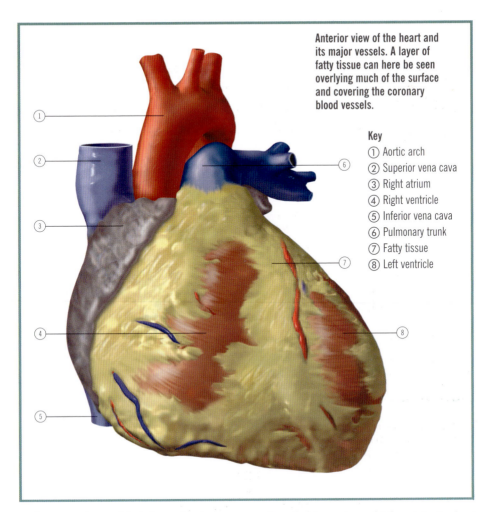

Anterior view of the heart and its major vessels. A layer of fatty tissue can here be seen overlying much of the surface and covering the coronary blood vessels.

**Key**
1. Aortic arch
2. Superior vena cava
3. Right atrium
4. Right ventricle
5. Inferior vena cava
6. Pulmonary trunk
7. Fatty tissue
8. Left ventricle

major, trapezius, and latissimus dorsi muscles; these afford some protection to the ribcage, as well as assisting in trunk and shoulder movement.

The pectoralis major and latissimus dorsi muscles act in two ways: in shoulder and arm movement or, when the arms are held fixed, to lift the chest (the pectorals) or bring the trunk forward (the latissimus). Not only does the trapezius participate in shoulder motion, it also plays a part in head movement when the shoulder is fixed. Numerous other muscles connected to the scapula act in shoulder and arm movement; those arising on the thoracic ribs include the pectoralis minor

and serratus anterior, which originates in a "sawtooth" pattern of piecewise attachments to individual ribs.

## Deep muscles

Deep, smaller muscles include the interspinals, which stabilize the vertebral column, and the intercostals. The intercostals connect the lower border of each rib to the upper border of the rib below. External intercostals spread the ribs, assisting in inspiration. Beneath the external muscles, and oriented at right angles to them, lie the internal intercostals, which pull the ribs together, causing forced expiration.

# THE ABDOMEN

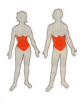

BETWEEN THE DIAPHRAGM AND PELVIC FLOOR is a large internal space called the abdominopelvic cavity. Its upper, abdominal spaces enclose the liver, spleen, gallbladder, pancreas, intestines, and kidneys; the lower, pelvic section contains the reproductive organs and urinary bladder.

## The peritoneum

Serous membrane linings define the abdominopelvic cavity's compartmental arrangement—as with organs in the thorax. Within the cavity is an extensive sac called the peritoneum. The sac's inner membrane secretes a serous fluid and the inner surfaces slide freely upon themselves. The outer surface is rougher, connective tissue that readily attaches to itself or to other tissues. The entire sac is sealed (in males) and empty but for its lubricants and lymph; it intrudes itself into spaces between and around many of the abdominopelvic organs. The **parietal peritoneum** attaches to the cavity surfaces, particularly at the front, sides, and diaphragm above, forming a lining for much of the abdominopelvic space and an anchor for holding everything in place.

The **visceral peritoneum** covers, envelops, or adheres to interior organs. To wrap partially or completely around an organ, the sac must generally be gathered into a fold or pleat, so peritoneal layers are often in contact with one another and with the organs or vessels enshrouded

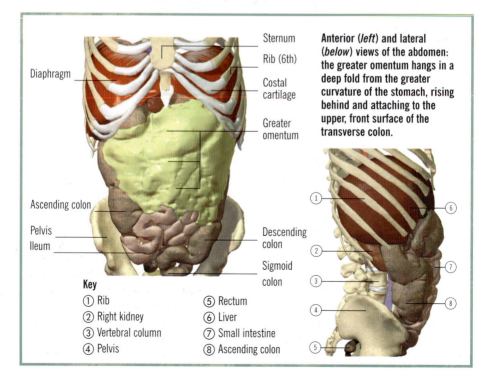

Diaphragm

Ascending colon

Pelvis

Ileum

Sternum

Rib (6th)

Costal cartilage

Greater omentum

Descending colon

Sigmoid colon

Anterior (*left*) and lateral (*below*) views of the abdomen: the greater omentum hangs in a deep fold from the greater curvature of the stomach, rising behind and attaching to the upper, front surface of the transverse colon.

**Key**

① Rib
② Right kidney
③ Vertebral column
④ Pelvis
⑤ Rectum
⑥ Liver
⑦ Small intestine
⑧ Ascending colon

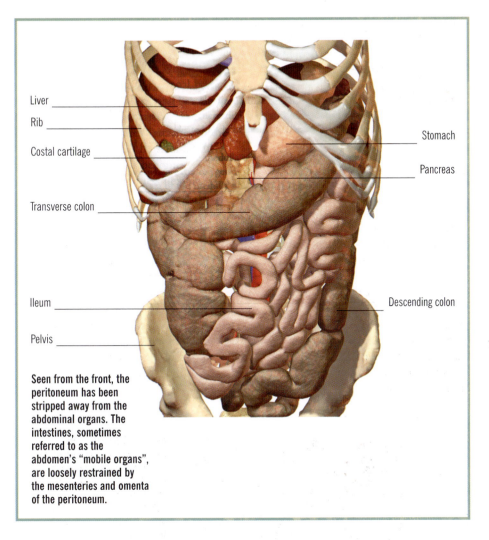

Liver

Rib

Costal cartilage

Transverse colon

Ileum

Pelvis

Stomach

Pancreas

Descending colon

**Seen from the front, the peritoneum has been stripped away from the abdominal organs. The intestines, sometimes referred to as the abdomen's "mobile organs", are loosely restrained by the mesenteries and omenta of the peritoneum.**

between them. Several abdominopelvic organs, e.g., the kidneys, bladder, pancreas, and most of the duodenum, are at most only partially surrounded by the peritoneum (i.e., **retroperitoneal**).

**Mesenteries** are peritoneal folds that enclose segments of the intestines and anchor them to the abdominal wall. Similar peritoneal folds, but connecting the stomach and other viscera, are the greater and lesser **omenta**. A mesentery's overlapped layers contain fat stores between them and carry nerves, blood, and lymph vessels that serve enclosed organs.

From shortly after conception, fetal mesenteric structures interact in a complex way with the fetal foregut, midgut, and hindgut to become differentiated segments of the alimentary canal. The origin of the digestive system is marked by the appearance of a single closed pouch, the primitive gut. It does not become continuous with openings at the mouth and anus until the eighth week. In time, through subsequent pouchings and specialization, the simple precursor segments become the entire digestive system and its accessory organs.

# THE ABDOMEN

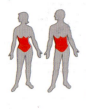

THE MUSCULAR WALLS OF THE ABDOMINOPELVIC cavity are principally formed, in front, by the rectus abdominus; at the sides, by a triple-layered group, the external oblique, internal oblique, and transversus abdominis; and, at the back, by the quadratus lumborum.

## The liver and spleen

A crescent-shaped fold, the **falciform ligament**, attaches the liver to the front of the abdominal wall and to part of the diaphragm. The left triangular ligament completes the diaphragm connection for the liver's left lobe; the coronary ligament of the liver does the same for the right lobe, though not all of that is covered by peritoneum—the liver has a triangular "bare area" at the back of its right lobe. The spleen is completely enwrapped in peritoneal folds, except at its **hilus**, where blood vessels enter.

## The stomach

To the left of centreline, and lying above the transverse colon, the stomach has a long, convex arc to its underside, its greater curvature. Its upper, concave surface is the lesser curvature. The greater **omentum** hangs in a thick fold from the greater curvature and duodenum to the transverse colon, where it joins with part of the **mesocolon**. As well as fat, these peritoneal folds are well supplied with lymph vessels, helping prevent infection. The lesser omentum extends between the lesser curvature and liver.

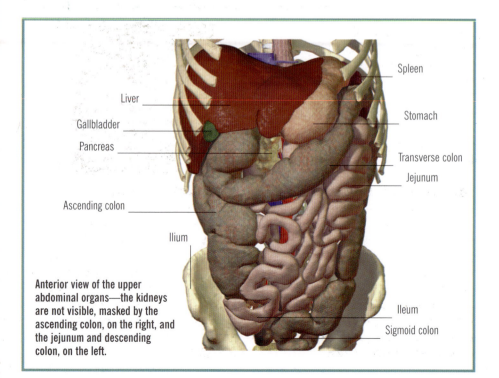

Spleen

Liver

Gallbladder

Pancreas

Stomach

Transverse colon

Jejunum

Ascending colon

Ilium

Ileum

Sigmoid colon

**Anterior view of the upper abdominal organs—the kidneys are not visible, masked by the ascending colon, on the right, and the jejunum and descending colon, on the left.**

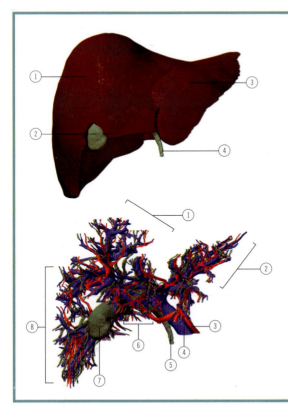

The liver in isolation (*top left*); stripping away its parenchyma (functional tissue) reveals a dense tracery (*bottom left*) of vascular and biliary vessels. An interior view of the gallbladder (*bottom right*) shows folds in its lining.

**Key (*top*)**
① Right lobe of liver
② Gallbladder
③ Left lobe of liver
④ Common bile duct

**Key (*bottom*)**
① Caudate brr
② Left brr
③ Proper hepatic artery
④ Portal vein
⑤ Common bile duct
⑥ Quadrate brr
⑦ Gallbladder
⑧ Right brr

# The small intestine

The **mesentery** of the small intestine fans out in sections from the posterior abdominal wall to suspend portions of the jejunum and ileum. Major blood vessels, the mesenteric artery and mesenteric vein (carrying absorbed nutrients), reach the intestines through the mesenteric structure.

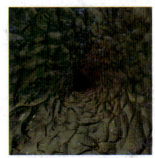

# The large intestine

Some diversity exists in the development of the large intestine's mesentery, the mesocolon. For most people, only the transverse and sigmoid colon are completely enfolded and connected to the abdominal wall, but sometimes additional mesenteric folds surround the ascending or descending colon. More usually, the ascending and descending segments are **retroperitoneal**.

# The pelvic region

The large bony girdle of the pelvis protects the organs contained in this area, and several muscles form a pelvic floor. Most of this cavity is enveloped in the **parietal peritoneum** membrane (though the bladder is not), but details are anatomically distinct in males and females. In females, peritoneal folds support the reproductive organs and the vagina.

# THE ARM AND HAND

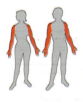

THE ARM AND HAND MAKE up what is perhaps the most flexible, versatile bony appendage in the animal kingdom. From the humerus to the tip of the little finger, the limb comprises 30 bones and a system of joints that includes examples of 6 different types of articular operation.

## The bones

The upper arm has only one bone, the humerus. **Distally**, the humerus has a complex double-condyle termination: **medially**, it receives the head of the ulna, the olecranon, and forms a hinge; **laterally**, a protuberance articulates with a concavity in the radius head to make an ellipsoidal joint. The ulna and radius also articulate with one another in two pivot joints.

At their distal ends, the ulna and radius form an ellipsoidal (condyloid) joint with

the wrist. Eight irregularly shaped but mutually fitted carpals form the wrist; each has limited freedom to slide on adjoining surfaces, in plane joints. Somewhat freer plane joints link the wrist to the last four metacarpals. That of the thumb articulates in a saddle joint with the trapezium, a wrist bone. Finger joints, at metacarpal distal ends and between phalanges, are condyloid. The thumb has only two phalangeal joints, as it lacks a middle bone.

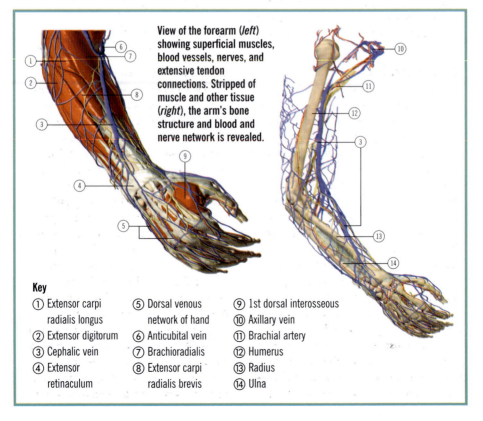

View of the forearm (*left*) showing superficial muscles, blood vessels, nerves, and extensive tendon connections. Stripped of muscle and other tissue (*right*), the arm's bone structure and blood and nerve network is revealed.

**Key**

1. Extensor carpi radialis longus
2. Extensor digitorum
3. Cephalic vein
4. Extensor retinaculum
5. Dorsal venous network of hand
6. Anticubital vein
7. Brachioradialis
8. Extensor carpi radialis brevis
9. 1st dorsal interosseous
10. Axillary vein
11. Brachial artery
12. Humerus
13. Radius
14. Ulna

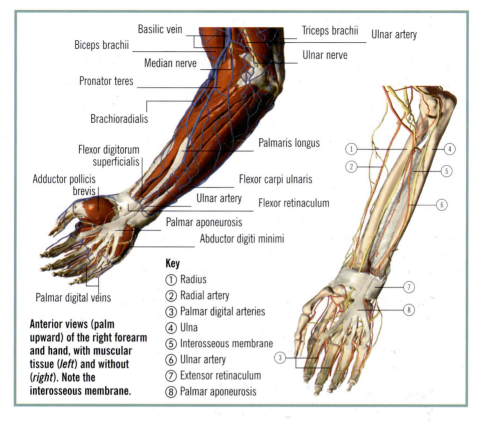

Basilic vein
Biceps brachii
Median nerve
Pronator teres
Brachioradialis
Flexor digitorum superficialis
Adductor pollicis brevis
Palmar aponeurosis
Abductor digiti minimi
Palmar digital veins

Triceps brachii    Ulnar artery
Ulnar nerve
Palmaris longus
Flexor carpi ulnaris
Ulnar artery    Flexor retinaculum

**Anterior views (palm upward) of the right forearm and hand, with muscular tissue (*left*) and without (*right*). Note the interosseous membrane.**

**Key**
1. Radius
2. Radial artery
3. Palmar digital arteries
4. Ulna
5. Interosseous membrane
6. Ulnar artery
7. Extensor retinaculum
8. Palmar aponeurosis

## The muscles

Altogether, nine muscles cross the shoulder joint to insert on the humerus. Among them, the prime movers of the arm are the deltoid, latissimus dorsi, and pectoralis major. Four rotator cuff muscles stabilize the shoulder joint.

One set of muscles that crosses the elbow joint either flexes or extends the forearm. An anterior group, the biceps brachii, brachialis, and brachioradialis, flexes the joint; posterior muscles, the triceps brachii and anconeus, extend it. Other muscles arise near the elbow joint, some attaching both at points on the humerus and ulna; these are mostly **extensors** and **flexors**, running the length of the forearm to insertions at the metacarpals. Together with others **originating** on the radius and ulna, they move the wrist and hand. Palmar muscles shape the palm;

three thenar (mound of the thumb) muscles—among several acting on the thumb—provide strength and the unusual opposability of the thumb. Subtle, fine movements are enabled by smaller muscles—seven interosseal and five lumbrical—acting on individual fingers.

## Blood and nerve supply

The axillary artery is the main supply vessel to the arm; its continuation into the arm, the brachial artery, divides just below the elbow into the radial and ulnar arteries. Venous blood in the hand and arm returns by way of five main veins, two deep and three superficial.

Five major nerves supply the arm and hand. One, the axillary nerve, serves only the upper limb. The others—the musculocutaneous, radial, median, and ulnar nerves—run the length of the arm.

# THE PELVIS

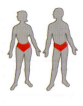

THE PELVIS PROVIDES A "FLOOR" FOR the abdominopelvic compartment above and a strong bony support for the torso. The lower limbs are attached here, at the hip; many blood vessels and nerves pass through and around the pelvic outlet, supplying the large muscles of the thigh and leg.

A basinlike assemblage of bones forms the pelvic girdle: at the centre is the sacrum and coccyx. The ossified contact surfaces between the sacrum and the iliac bones link the tower of the axial skeleton to its lower-limb locomotion. The iliac bones sweep around the sides of the pelvic region and unite with other pairs, the ischium and pubic bones, forming the acetabulum. At the front, the medial ends of the left and right pubic bones come together at the pubic symphysis.

The broad iliac surfaces provide **origin** for numerous hip and thigh muscles, among them the gluteals, iliacus, sartorius, tensor fasciae latae, and rectus femoris. Others, arising from ischial or pubic surfaces of the pelvis, include the gracilus, semimembranosus, semitendinosus, pectineus, obturators and thigh adductors. Lower back muscles and the muscle sheets surrounding the abdominopelvic cavity also have attachment to the sacral or iliac upper borders: the erector spinae, quadratus lumborum, lattissimus dorsi, external oblique, and transversus abdominis. The rectus abdominis attaches at it lower end to the pubic symphysis.

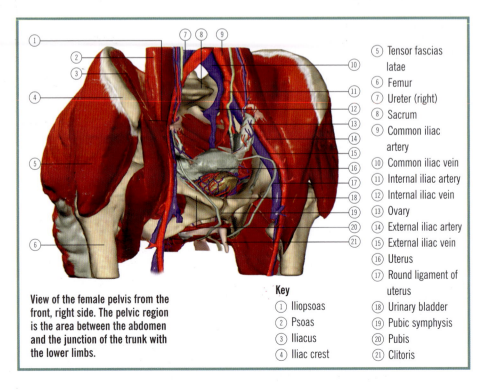

View of the female pelvis from the front, right side. The pelvic region is the area between the abdomen and the junction of the trunk with the lower limbs.

**Key**

1. Iliopsoas
2. Psoas
3. Iliacus
4. Iliac crest
5. Tensor fascias latae
6. Femur
7. Ureter (right)
8. Sacrum
9. Common iliac artery
10. Common iliac vein
11. Internal iliac artery
12. Internal iliac vein
13. Ovary
14. External iliac artery
15. External iliac vein
16. Uterus
17. Round ligament of uterus
18. Urinary bladder
19. Pubic symphysis
20. Pubis
21. Clitoris

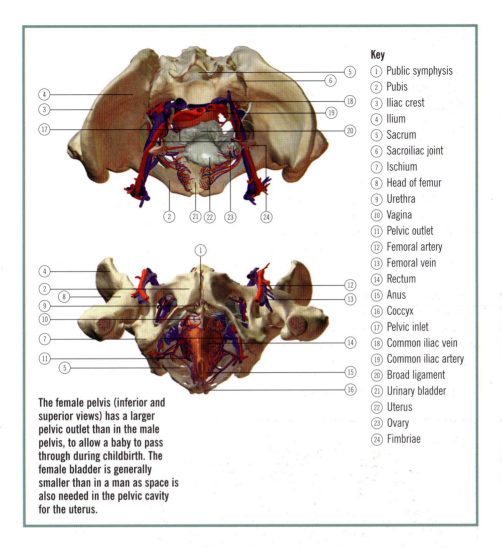

**Key**
1. Public symphysis
2. Pubis
3. Iliac crest
4. Ilium
5. Sacrum
6. Sacroiliac joint
7. Ischium
8. Head of femur
9. Urethra
10. Vagina
11. Pelvic outlet
12. Femoral artery
13. Femoral vein
14. Rectum
15. Anus
16. Coccyx
17. Pelvic inlet
18. Common iliac vein
19. Common iliac artery
20. Broad ligament
21. Urinary bladder
22. Uterus
23. Ovary
24. Fimbriae

The female pelvis (inferior and superior views) has a larger pelvic outlet than in the male pelvis, to allow a baby to pass through during childbirth. The female bladder is generally smaller than in a man as space is also needed in the pelvic cavity for the uterus.

A slinglike pelvic floor is created by layers of muscles, some of which also function in defecation and urination; these are the levator ani and coccygeus, making up the pelvic diaphragm. Lower down, the deep transverse perineus and urethral sphincter, together with the tough perineal membrane, form the urogenital diaphragm.

Like the abdominal space above and continuous with it, the pelvic cavity is lined by the peritoneum. The urinary bladder, which rests on the pelvic floor, is covered by the peritoneum only on its upper surface—which helps hold it in place—and it is, thus, **retroperitoneal**. The female reproductive organs, the uterus and ovaries, are held in peritoneal folds of the broad ligament.

Major blood vessels, the external iliac artery and vein, leave the pelvic region by passing in front of the pubis and descending along the femur's medial side. The organs and tissue of the pelvis are mostly supplied by the internal iliac artery, the smaller branch of the common iliac artery. The body's largest nerve, the sciatic nerve, passes through the pelvic outlet into the lower limb, as does the femoral nerve.

# THE LEG AND FOOT

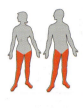

THE THIGH, LEG, AND FOOT FORM the means of typical human locomotion. Their joints are less flexible than those of the arm, and their muscles are larger. Instead of fanning into supple digits, the leg terminates in a sort of springy shock absorber—the structures of the foot.

## The bones

The femur carries the upper body's weight from the hip joint to the knee joint. In front of the knee is the triangular patella. From knee to ankle, weight is borne by the tibia, with some support contributed by the more slender fibula.

The ankle is structured from seven irregularly shaped bones, the tarsals. The largest, the calcaneus, or heel-bone, has a thick backward projection that provides a lever for the calf muscles used in **plantar flexion**. A central pivot, the talus, forms

condyloid joints with the tibia and fibula above, calcaneus below, and navicular bone in front of it. The remaining, distal tarsals articulate with 5 metatarsal bones, and these articulate with the 14 phalanges of the toes. Just as with the thumb, the great toe (hallux), has only two phalanges.

## The muscles

The powerful thigh muscles originate in the pelvis, cross the hip joint and insert into the femur or continue across the

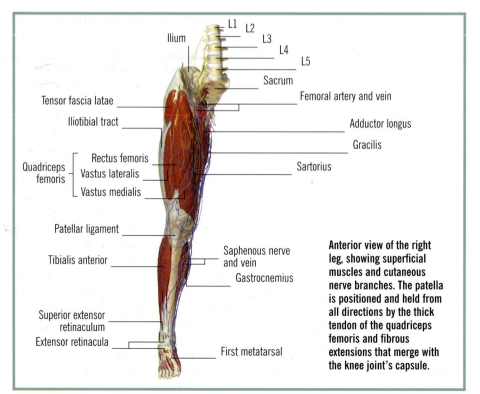

Ilium
L1 L2 L3 L4 L5
Sacrum
Tensor fascia latae
Femoral artery and vein
Iliotibial tract
Adductor longus
Gracilis
Rectus femoris
Quadriceps femoris
Vastus lateralis
Vastus medialis
Sartorius
Patellar ligament
Tibialis anterior
Saphenous nerve and vein
Gastrocnemius
Superior extensor retinaculum
Extensor retinacula
First metatarsal

**Anterior view of the right leg, showing superficial muscles and cutaneous nerve branches. The patella is positioned and held from all directions by the thick tendon of the quadriceps femoris and fibrous extensions that merge with the knee joint's capsule.**

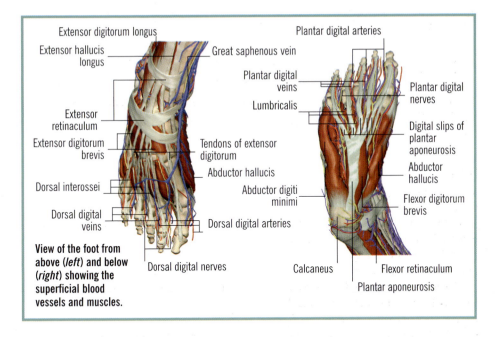

Extensor digitorum longus

Extensor hallucis longus

Great saphenous vein

Plantar digital arteries

Plantar digital veins

Lumbricalis

Plantar digital nerves

Extensor retinaculum

Extensor digitorum brevis

Tendons of extensor digitorum

Abductor hallucis

Digital slips of plantar aponeurosis

Abductor hallucis

Dorsal interossei

Abductor digiti minimi

Flexor digitorum brevis

Dorsal digital veins

Dorsal digital arteries

**View of the foot from above (*left*) and below (*right*) showing the superficial blood vessels and muscles.**

Dorsal digital nerves

Calcaneus

Flexor retinaculum

Plantar aponeurosis

knee joint, to attach at the tibia. Anterior thigh muscles flex the thigh; the quadriceps femoris is the prime mover. Posterior muscles, principally the hamstrings, extend the thigh and cross the knee joint to flex the knee. **Adductors**, in the medial thigh, pull the leg inward, to the centreline; these include the gracilis, pectineus, and the adductors brevis, longus, and magnus. Most also assist the quadriceps in **flexion**. The long, straplike sartorius is an **abductor**, as are the gluteal muscles, of the posterior pelvis and thigh. The lower leg muscles arise on the tibia and fibula, with the exception of the gastrocnemius, which originates in the distal femur.

Anterior muscles, such as the tibialis anterior and extensor digitorum longus, **dorsiflex** the foot, bending it upward at the ankle. The extensor digitorum longus also extends the toes. Posterior muscles plantar flex the foot, bending it downward. Lateral muscles, the peroneals, plantar flex the foot and turn it outward. Within the foot itself, smaller, intrinsic

muscles are held in a web of tendons radiating from the plantar **aponeurosis**.

## Blood and nerve supply

The thigh muscles receive blood through the external iliac artery and its continuation as it enters the thigh, the femoral artery. Just above the knee the femoral becomes the popliteal artery, which branches below the knee into the anterior and posterior tibial arteries. The anterior tibial artery continues into the foot as the dorsal pedis artery, dividing into lateral tarsal, medial tarsal, and arcuate branches. The posterior tibial artery gives rise to a major offshoot, the peroneal artery, before dividing at the ankle into medial and lateral plantar arteries.

Nerves to the thigh, leg, and foot originate in the lumbar and sacral plexuses. Those from the lumbar plexus include the femoral nerve, the obturator nerve, and the lateral femoral cutaneous. Arising from the sacral plexus are the sciatic nerve, superior and inferior gluteal nerves, and the posterior femoral cutaneous.

# GLOSSARY

**Abduction**   Movement of a bone or limb away from the midline of the body.

**Absorption**   The process of absorbing simple nutrient molecules into the bloodstream.

**Acini**   Cell clusters within the pancreas that secrete digestive juice.

**Actin**   One of two proteins constituting the myofilament of muscle.

**Adduction**   Movement of a limb or bone towards the midline of the body (opposite of **abduction**).

**Adipose**   Relating to fat.

**Adrenaline**   *See* **epinephrine**.

**Adrenocorticotropic hormone** (**ACTH**)   Hormone produced by the anterior pituitary gland in response to corticotropin-releasing hormone, produced by the hypothalamus. ACTH stimulates the adrenals to produce various steroid hormones.

**Afferent**   Towards a centre; usually relating to arteries, veins, or nerves; e.g., afferent nerves carry input from sensory receptors to the central nervous system.

**Agonist**   Prime mover; a muscle that provides the main force for a movement.

**Aldosterone**   Hormone produced by the adrenal cortex that causes sodium retention by the kidneys.

**Alpha cell**   Cells within the pancreatic islets of the pancreas that release the hormone glucagon, in response to low glucose levels. Glucagon stimulates the liver to turn glycogen into glucose.

**Amniotic fluid**   Protective fluid filling the amnion, the membrane surrounding the fetus, in which the fetus is free to move.

**Ampulla**   A small dilation in a canal or duct.

**Amylase**   Enzyme found in saliva that breaks down starch into maltose.

**Anastomosis**   Area where two branching communications networks, e.g., nerves, arteries, or blood vessels, join.

**Androgen**   Male sex steroid hormone. The principal mammalian androgen is testosterone.

**Antagonist**   A muscle that opposes the action of a prime mover (e.g., the triceps brachii—the prime mover of forearm extension—is the antagonist of the biceps brachii—the prime mover of forearm flexion).

**Anterior**   Before; in front of; in the front part of; anatomical term referring to the front part of the body, or of any structure; opposite of **posterior**. *See also* **ventral**.

**Antibody**   Proteins produced by lymphocytes in response to an antigen (such as a toxin or bacteria), which the antibody then destroys.

**Antidiuretic hormone** (**ADH**)   Hormone secreted by the posterior pituitary gland. Causes the kidneys to retain water, thus secreting more concentrated urine.

**Aponeuroses**   Flat, straplike tendons that link muscle to bone and also muscle to muscle.

**Artery**   A blood vessel that carries blood away from the heart.

**Atrial systole**   Contraction of the two atria during the cardiac cycle, causing them to empty of blood and consequently filling the ventricles.

**Atrioventricular valve**   A valve within the heart that allows blood to flow in one direction only, from atria to ventricles.

**Axial hair**   Secondary hair growth (armpit hair).

**Axon**   The electrical impulse-carrying process of a nerve cell.

**Bacteria**   Unicellular (single-celled) organisms that have an outer coating, the cell wall, in addition to a plasma membrane; do not have a nucleus or other membrane-bound organelles.

**Biconvex**   A lens that is convex on both sides.

**Bile**   A yellowish brown/green alkaline fluid secreted by the liver. It is discharged into the duodenum where it aids in the digestion of fats.

**Binocular vision**   Three-dimensional vision.

**Bipennate**   A pennate muscle where fascicles are attached to both sides of the central tendon like a feather (e.g., rectus femoris).

**B-lymphocyte**   A specialized lymphocyte that produces antibodies to a specific antigen.

**Bone marrow**   Soft tissue filling the porous cavity of the bone shaft. Red marrow found in the ribs, vertebrae, pelvis, and skull produces blood cells; yellow marrow found in the centre of long bones consists of fatty material.

**Broad ligament**   Fold of peritoneum that supports the uterus, uterine tubes, and vagina.

**Brush border enzyme**   Enzymes attached to microvilli in the small intestine.

**Calcitonin**, *thyrocalcitonin*   Hormone secreted by the parathyroid glands; decreases blood calcium levels by inhibiting bone resorption.

**Calyces**   Small cup-shaped cavities in the kidneys formed from the branching of the renal pelvis; they cover the tips of the medullary pyramids and collect urine.

**Capillaries**   Tiny blood vessels that link the arterial and venous systems.

**Carboxypeptidase**   Enzyme found in pancreatic juice that breaks down proteins.

**Cardiac cycle**   The heartbeat; a regulated cycle of events that causes the heart to beat; includes systole (contraction) and diastole (relaxation).

**Cardioacceleratory centre**   Area of the medulla oblongata in the brain stem responsible for accelerating the heart rate when extra oxygen is needed.

**Cardioinhibitory centre**   Area of the medulla oblongata in the brainstem responsible for slowing the heart rate when the body is at rest.

**Cartilage**   Specialized connective tissue found at joints; provides support and aids movement.

**Catalyst**   Substance that speeds up a chemical reaction.

**Caudal**   Anatomical term relating to the tail end. *See also* **inferior**.

**Cellulose**   Polysaccharide sugar; the major nutritional constituent of grass, hay, and leaves; it forms the major energy source for herbivorous mammals.

**Cerebrospinal fluid**   Clear fluid, similar to blood plasma; fills the ventricles of the brain, and the space surrounding the brain and spinal cord.

**Cervical vertebrae**   Seven small bones of the spine that form the neck.

**Cholecystokinin**   A digestive hormone secreted from the wall of the duodenum; it causes contraction of the gallbladder and the subsequent release of bile into, and along, the common bile duct where it is released into the duodenum.

**Chyme**   Semi-liquid paste produced from food by the action of gastric juice and the crushing action of the stomach.

**Chymotrypsin**   Enzyme found in pancreatic juice that breaks down proteins.

**Cilia**   Microscopic hairlike processes; produce a rhythmic paddling motion, extending from the surface of many cell types. *See also* **flagellum**.

**Circumvallate papillae**   The largest of the papillae, to be found at the rear of the tongue; contain taste buds.

**Collagen**   Tough, fibrous protein found in bone fibres, cartilage, and connective tissue.

**Concave**   A surface that is depressed or hollowed.

**Conchae**   A shell-shaped structure projecting from the lateral wall of the nasal cavity.

**Cones**   One of two types of photoreceptor cells found in the retina; very sensitive to colour but unable to detect light at very faint levels.

**Convex**   A surface that is evenly curved or bulging outward.

**Core body temperature**   The temperature of the inner body—the organs—as opposed to that of the skin.

**Coronal**   Relating to a corona or crown.

**Corpus cavernosa** ("cavernous body")   One of two parallel columns of erectile tissue in the penis.

**Corpus spongiosum** ("spongy body")   Median column of erectile tissue located between the corpus cavernosa; terminates as the enlarged glans penis and is traversed by the urethra.

**Corticosteroid**   Steroid hormones produced by the adrenal cortex. There are three groups: glucocorticoids, mineralocorticoids, and gonadocorticoids.

**Cortisol**   Glucocorticoid hormone; stabilizes blood glucose levels and has anti-inflammatory action.

**Coxal**   Of, or relating to, the hip.

**Cranial**   Relating to the cranium or head; anatomical term referring to anything headward. *See also* **superior**.

**Cupula**   A cup-shaped or domelike structure; the domelike end of the cochlea.

**Dendrites**   Branched processes that carry nerve impulses towards the cell body.

**Depression**   A downward movement; opposite of **elevation**; a movement that flattens or lowers a body part.

**Diaphysis**   Bone shaft; composed of compact bone.

**Diastole**  The dilation of the atria and the ventricles during the cardiac cycle, causing the atria to fill with blood.

**Diffusion**  A passive-transport mechanism. The movement of molecules from an area of high concentration into an area of low concentration until the two are evenly balanced.

**Digestion**  Breakdown of foods into simpler nutrient molecules.

**Distal**  Situated away from the centre of the body; anatomical term usually referring to an extremity or distant part of a limb or organ.

**Dorsal**  Relating to the back, or back part of the body or organ. *See also* **posterior**.

**Dorsiflexion**  Flexion of the foot (bending upwards).

**Ductus arteriosus**  A blood vessel in the fetus that connects the left pulmonary artery with the abdominal aorta; allows fetal blood to bypass the nonfunctioning fetal lungs.

**Effector**  A tissue complex capable of an effective response to the stimulus of a nervous impulse.

**Egestion**  Elimination of undigested food.

**Ejaculation**  The expulsion or emission of semen through the penis via the urethra.

**Elastin**  The major fibrous connective tissue protein found in elastic structures.

**Elevation**  A movement that raises a body part; lifting upward; opposite of **depression**.

**Endochondral**  Situated within, or taking place within cartilage.

**Endocrine**  Secreting into the bloodstream; usually refers to a gland that produces a secretion (such as a hormone) that circulates in the blood to act upon a distant organ or gland.

**Endothelium**  A layer of smooth, flat cells lining blood and lymphatic vessels; inner mucous membrane lining the uterus.

**Enzyme**  A protein that acts as a biological catalyst.

**Epimysium**  A sheath of connective tissue binding groups of muscle fascicles.

**Epinephrine**, *adrenaline*  Hormone secreted by the adrenal medulla in response to stimulation by the autonomic nervous system. It increases metabolic rates in preparation for "fight or flight".

**Epineurium**  Outer connective tissue sheath surrounding bundles of nerve fascicles and the nerve's blood vessels.

**Epiphysis**  Extremity (bone end); composed of spongy bone tissue.

**Erythropoietin**  Hormone released by the kidneys. It stimulates the production of red blood cells.

**Evert**  Turning the sole of the foot outward; opposite of **invert**.

**Exocrine**  Glandular secretion that is delivered to a surface through a duct.

**Extension**  An increase in the angle of a joint (opposite of **flexion**).

**Extracellular**  Outside cells.

**Falciform ligament**  A crescent-shaped fold of peritoneum that extends from the diaphragm to the liver and anchors the liver to the anterior wall of the abdomen.

**Fascicle**  A bundle of muscle or nerve fibres.

**Feces**  Semi-solid, undigested matter that is stored in the large intestine until such time as it is excreted; consists of undigested food, epithelium, intestinal mucus, and bacteria.

**Feedback mechanism**  The return, as input, of output of a given system; functions as a regulatory mechanism.

**Fetus**  An unborn embryo after 13 weeks' development; the unborn young of a mammal that has taken form in the uterus; the product of conception.

**Fibrin**  The insoluble, stringy plasma protein that forms the essential part of a blood clot.

**Fibrinogen**  The inactive form of a coagulative protein; it is converted into insoluble fibrin during clot formation.

**Filiform papillae**  Pointed papillae covering the surface of the tongue. The most numerous of the papillae, they give the tongue its rough surface.

**Fixator**  A synergist that provides a stable origin for the action of the prime mover.

**Flagellum** (pl. **flagella**)  A whiplike appendage of certain cells; used for locomotory purposes to propel a cell through a fluid environment; a whiplike, locomotory organelle.

**Flatus**  Gas produced by anaerobic bacteria in the large intestine.

**Flexion**  A decrease in the angle of a joint; opposite of **extension**.

**Follicle**  A small sac or secretory cavity.

**Follicle-stimulating hormone** (**FSH**)  Hormone secreted by the anterior pituitary gland; stimulates egg maturation and oestrogen release in the ovary, and testosterone production.

**Foramen**   A natural opening or hole through a bone.

**Foramen ovale** ("oval opening")   The hole between the two atria in the fetal heart, diverting approximately one-third of the blood that arrives in the right atrium directly into the left atrium.

**Foregut**   The upper (cranial) portion of the primitive alimentary canal in the embryo; eventually forms the oesophagus, stomach, duodenum, liver, and pancreas.

**Fulcrum**   The point on which a lever turns.

**Fundus**   Upper region of the stomach.

**Fungiform papillae**   Mushroom-shaped papillae scattered irregularly over the surface of the tongue; contain taste buds.

**Ganglion**   A swelling at the junction between the preganglionic and postganglionic neurons.

**Gastric pits**   Depressions within the lining of the stomach; contain glands that produce stomach acid (gastric juice).

**Glans**   A conical acorn-shaped structure (often refers to the glans penis, the conical extension of the corpus spongiosum forming the head of the penis).

**Glomerular capsule**   Cup-shaped end of the renal tubule.

**Glomerulus**   Mass of blood capillaries within the nephron of the kidney.

**Glucagon**   Hormone produced by the pancreas that promotes the conversion of glycogen into glucose.

**Glucocorticoid**   Corticosteroids produced by the adrenals; important in protein and carbohydrate metabolism.

**Glucose**   A simple sugar, very important in metabolism and the principle source of energy for the brain.

**Glycogen**   A polysaccharide broken down by glucagon into glucose; the principal carbohydrate reserve.

**Gonadocorticoid**   Androgens or male sex hormones.

**Gonadotropic hormones**   Hormones (luteinizing hormone and follicle-stimulating hormone) released from the pituitary; influence the activity of the gonads.

**Granulocyte**   A white blood cell; it detects, surrounds, engulfs, and digests pathogens.

**Growth hormone (GH)**   Hormone secreted by the anterior pituitary gland; stimulates growth during childhood and adolescence, and converts glycogen into glucose.

**Gyrus (pl. gyri)**   A convolution (ridge) in the cortex of the cerebral hemisphere of the brain, separated by sulci.

**Haemoglobin**   The globular iron-containing protein found in red blood cells; responsible for oxygen and carbon dioxide transport.

**Haustra**   The pouches or bulges in the colon formed by the uneven pull of the teniae coli.

**Hepatocyte**   A liver cell.

**Hilus**   A small indent or depression in an organ where arteries, veins, and nerves enter and leave.

**Hindgut**   The caudal or terminal portion of the embryonic alimentary canal; eventually forms the large intestine, rectum, and anal canal.

**Homeostasis**   The state of balance and stability that exist inside a healthy body regardless of changes in the internal and external environments.

**Hormone**   Chemicals synthesized and secreted by endocrine glands into the bloodstream; may have local or general effects.

**Hydrolysis**   The splitting of a compound by the addition of water.

**Ileocaecal valve**   Valve separating the ileum from the large intestine.

**Inferior**   Lower; below, in relation to another structure. *See also* **caudal**.

**Ingestion**   Process by which food is taken into the body.

**Insertion**   The end of a muscle to which is attached a moving bone.

**Inspiratory centre**   Area of the brainstem that controls breathing rate and depth.

**Insulin**   Pancreatic hormone that regulates sugar levels; facilitates the conversion of glucose into glycogen.

**Interstitial cells,** *Leydig cells*   Cells of the testes that produce testosterone on stimulation with luteinizing hormone.

**Interstitial fluid**   Fluid found between cells that bathes and nourishes surrounding body tissues.

**Intervertebral disc**   Jellylike cartilaginous pad that lies between each vertebra.

**Intracellular**   Inside cells.

**Intramembranous**   Inside membrane.

**Invert**   Turning the sole of the foot inward; opposite of **evert**.

**Islets of Langerhans**   Microscopic endocrine cells of the pancreas. There are three types: alpha cells secrete glucagon; beta cells secrete insulin; and delta cells secrete gastrin.

**Isometric contraction**   Muscle contraction whereby tension develops and the muscle exerts a pulling force, but does not shorten due to opposing forces.

**Isotonic contraction**   Muscle contraction whereby the muscle contracts and gets shorter, causing movement.

**Keratin**   A tough protein that forms the outer layer of hair and nails; it is soft in hair and hard in nails.

**Lactase**   The enzyme that breaks down lactose (milk sugar) into glucose and galactose in the small intestine.

**Lacteal**   Lymphatic capillary network that extends into the villi of the small intestine.

**Lateral**   Away from the midline of the body (to the side).

**Leydig cells**   See *interstitial cells*.

**Libido**   Conscious or unconscious sexual desire. A term introduced by Freud.

**Lipase**   Enzyme found in pancreatic juice that breaks down fats.

**Lumbar vertebrae**   The five large bones that form the small of the back.

**Lumen**   The interior space within a tube-shaped structure or body.

**Luteinizing hormone** (**LH**)   Hormone secreted by the anterior pituitary gland. It stimulates ovulation and progesterone secretion in females, and testosterone secretion in males.

**Lymphocyte**   A white blood cell formed in lymphatic tissue; the main producer of antibodies.

**Macrophage**   Any large mononuclear phagocytic cell; may be wandering or fixed.

**Macula lutea**   The central area of the retina; contains cones only.

**Maltase**   Brush-border enzyme found in pancreatic juice; breaks down maltose into glucose.

**Mammary gland**   The breast; rounded eminence composed mainly of adipose (fat) and glandular tissue; produces milk during lactation.

**Median**   An anatomical term. Towards the midline of the body.

**Mediastinum**   The thin-walled cavity between the two lungs. It contains the oesophagus, trachea, blood, and lymphatic vessels, and also the pericardial cavity.

**Medullary pyramids**   Cone-shaped filtration units within the inner core of the kidney.

**Meninges**   The three protective tissue layers (dura mater, arachnoid mater, and pia mater) that surround and encase the brain and spinal cord.

**Menopause**   The cessation of the menstrual cycle in the mature female.

**Menstrual cycle**   The monthly cycle of events occurring between puberty and the menopause that prepares the uterus for pregnancy. If pregnancy does not occur, mucus, blood, and sloughed endometrial tissue discharge through the vagina.

**Mesentary**   Fused and folded layers of visceral peritoneum that attach abdominopelvic organs to the cavity wall.

**Mesocolon**   The fold of visceral peritoneum that attaches the colon to the posterior abdominal wall.

**Mesometrium**   Part of the broad and round ligaments; secures the uterus in the pelvic cavity.

**Metabolism**   The sum of all physical and chemical processes that occur in the body. May either build up or break down substances.

**Microvilli**   Microscopic hairlike projections lining the intestinal surface.

**Midgut**   The central portion of the alimentary canal in the embryo (small intestine); situated between the foregut and the hindgut;

**Mineralocorticoid**   A corticosteroid hormone secreted by the adrenal cortex. Maintains salt (sodium and potassium) levels.

**Mitral valve**   The left atrioventricular heart valve; also known as the bicuspid valve.

**Monochrome**   Single colour; images generated by the rods of the retina.

**Monocyte**   Mononuclear phagocytes formed in bone marrow and transported to tissues where they develop into macrophages.

**Motor neuron**   Carry motor output from the CNS to muscles and glands.

**Multipennate**   A pennate muscle with many bipennate units (e.g., deltoid).

**Myofibril**   Small fibres within a single muscle fibre. Each fibre is packed with thousands of myofibrils that run the entire length of the muscle fibre.

**Myoglobin**   The red pigment, similar to haemoglobin, that is found in muscles.

**Myometrium**   The middle, muscular layer of the uterus.

**Myosin**   A large protein that makes up the thick myofilaments of muscle fibres.

**Nephron**   The functional filtration unit of the kidney; each kidney contains millions of nephrons, all of which independently filter blood to produce urine.

**Nerve impulses**   Electrical signal that passes at high speed from one end of a nerve to another.

**Neurons**   Nerve cells.

**Neurotransmitter**   Chemical released from the synaptic knob of a neuron, which travels across the synapse generating a nerve impulse in the recipient neuron.

**Nipple**   Cylindrical or conical projection from just below the centre of the breast, from where glandular secretions (colostrum and breastmilk) are emitted.

**Nitrogenous**   Nitrogen-containing.

**Noradrenaline**   *See* **norepinephrine**.

**Norepinephrine**, *noradrenaline*   Hormone secreted by the adrenal medulla in response to stimulation by the autonomic nervous system. It increases metabolic rates in preparation for the "fight or flight" response.

**Nuclease**   Enzyme found in pancreatic juice that breaks down nucleic acids (such as DNA).

**Nucleus**   A large spherical membrane-bound cellular organelle; present in most cells, it contains most of the cell's DNA and RNA; a cluster of neuronal cell bodies in the CNS.

**Oestrogen**   Family of sex hormones produced by the ovaries. Cause maturation and maintenance of the female reproductive system; responsible for the development of secondary female sexual characteristics; prepares the body for pregnancy.

**Olfactory**   Pertaining to the sense of smell.

**Omentum** (pl. **omenta**)   The fold of peritoneum that encloses the main digestive organs and hangs like an apron in front of the intestines.

**Oocyte**   An immature ovum (egg).

**Opposition**   Movement of the thumb to touch (oppose) the tip of another finger.

**Organ of Corti**   The organ of hearing.

**Origin**   The end of a muscle attached to a bone that does not move.

**Osseous**   Bony.

**Ossicles**   The bones of the ear: the malleus (hammer), incus (anvil), and stapes (stirrup).

**Ossification**   The formation of bone from soft hyaline cartilage or fibrous membrane.

**Osteoblast**   Bone cell capable of forming new bone matrix; usually found on the growing portions of bones.

**Osteoclast**   A multinuclear cell capable of destroying bone; usually found at places of bone resorption.

**Osteocyte**   Bone cell found in mature bone tissue; helps to regulate calcium concentrations in the body by releasing calcium from bone into the blood. The principal type of cell found in bone.

**Osteon**   Concentric cylinder of calcified bone that makes up compact bone.

**Ovarian cycle**   The monthly cycle of events leading up to the release of a mature egg or ovum.

**Ovarian ligament**   Ligament that anchors each ovary medially to the uterus.

**Ovulation**   Monthly process in which a mature egg (ovum) is released from the ovary in preparation to be fertilized.

**Ovum**   An egg; the female sex cell.

**Oxytocin**   Hormone secreted by the pituitary; stimulates uterine contractions during labour and the release of breastmilk.

**Papillae**   Small projections on the upper surface of the tongue; there are several kinds, distinguished by their shapes (circumvallate, filiform, fungiform, lentiform) and most house taste buds.

**Parathormone**   *See* **parathyroid hormone**.

**Parathyroid hormone** (PTH), *parathormone*   Hormone released by the parathyroid glands; helps to raise blood calcium levels.

**Parietal peritoneum**   The serous membrane that lines the outer wall of the abdominal cavity.

**Pathogen**   A virus, microorganism, or other foreign substance that causes disease.

**Pennate muscle**   A muscle where the fascicles are arranged obliquely to a long tendon.

**Peptidase**   Brush border enzyme; breaks down peptides into amino acids.

**Pericardial cavity**   Fluid-filled cavity that lies between the pericardia, the serous membranes that cover the heart and line the thoracic cavity; allows the heart to contract without friction.

**Perimetrium**   Layer of visceral peritoneum that surrounds the uterus; the serous coat of the uterus.

**Perimysium**   A connective tissue sheath that binds each muscle fascicle.

**Perineurium**   Sheath of connective tissue surrounding each nerve fascicle.

**Periosteum**   Membrane that covers bone.

**Peripheral vision**   The outer edge of the visual field.

**Peristalsis**   Waves of successive muscle contractions and relaxations that push substances through biological tubes (e.g., food through the oesophagus, urine through the ureter).

**pH**   Measure of the acidity or alkalinity of a solution.

**Phagocyte**   A scavenger cell that engulfs and digests other cells, bacteria, microorganisms, or foreign matter.

**Photoreceptors**   Light-sensitive sensory receptors that are found in the retina.

**Placenta**   A thick spongy tissue bed containing a rich supply of blood vessels that forms in the wall of the uterus during pregnancy. It supplies nutrients to the fetus and in return collects waste material via the umbilical cord.

**Plantar flexion**   Extension (straightening) of the foot.

**Platelets**   A cell fragment found in blood that is important for blood clotting.

**Pleura** (pl. **pleurae**)   The serous membrane covering the lungs and lining the walls of the pleural cavity.

**Plicae circulares**   Circular folds in the small intestine that increase the available surface area for the absorption of nutrients.

**Porta hepatis**   Area of the liver, situated on the lower posterior surface, through which blood vessels, nerves, lymphatics, and ducts enter and leave the liver.

**Posterior**   Behind, after; opposite of **anterior**. *See also* **dorsal**.

**Postganglionic**   Referring to neurons arising at an autonomic ganglion and carrying nerve signals to smooth muscle, the heart, or glands (that is, to some part served by the autonomic nerve system (ANS).

**Preganglionic**   First neuron in a two-neuron chain of the ANS.

**Primary visual cortex**   Area of the brain (located in the occipital lobe) that perceives and interprets visual images.

**Prolactin**   Hormone that encourages breast tissue growth and milk production.

**Pronation**   A movement of the forearm that turns the palm downward; opposite of **supination**.

**Prostate**   A male secretory gland surrounding the urethra at the neck of the bladder. Its secretions reduce vaginal acidity and increase sperm motility.

**Proximal**   Situated nearer or towards the centre of the body (or attached end of a limb); anatomical term usually referring to a limb or organ; opposite of **distal**.

**Puberty**   The state of reaching sexual maturity. When one is capable of sexual reproduction.

**Pulmonary**   Pertaining to the lungs.

**Pulmonary circuit**   The circuit whereby deoxygenated blood is pumped by the right side of the heart to the lungs via the pulmonary artery. Oxygenated blood is returned to the left side of the heart via the pulmonary vein.

**Pylorus**   Funnel-shaped lower region of the stomach that links with the duodenum.

**Rectal valves**   Three transverse folds within the rectum that enable feces to be separated from flatus, enabling flatus to be voided without pushing out feces.

**Refraction**   The bending of light waves as they pass between two mediums of different densities.

**Releasing factor**   Hormone secreted by the hypothalamus that stimulates the release of pituitary hormones.

**Renal capsule**   One of three tissue layers that surrounds the kidney; a fibrous coat that helps to prevent the spread of infection into the kidney.

**Renal fascia**   The third and outermost tissue layer surrounding the kidney; it anchors it to the abdominal wall.

**Renal sinus**   Central recess within the kidney that follows on from the hilus; is continuous with the renal capsule and is almost entirely filled with the renal pelvis and renal vessels.

**Renal tubule**   Tube that loops between the cortex and medulla of the kidney (part of the nephron) and which empties into the renal pelvis through a collecting duct.

**Reposition**   Movement of the thumb away from the tip of another finger.

**Retinacula**   Flat, fibrous straps that hold tendons in place.

**Retroperitoneal**   Located external or posterior to the abdominopelvic cavity and the peritoneum.

**Rods**   One of two types of photoreceptor cells found in the retina; they are very sensitive to light but not to colour.

**Rostral**   Situated at, or directed towards the anterior end of an organism.

**Rotation**   A pivoting movement that twists a body part on its long axis; movement of a bone around its long axis.

**Rotator cuff muscles**   The four scapula muscles (supraspinatus, infraspinatus, teres minor, and subscapularis) that stabilize the shoulder joint.

**Rugae**   Folds or ridges within the lining of a tissue, such as the stomach or vagina.

**Saccule**   A small sac or pouch. The smaller of the two balance detectors in the vestibule of the ear.

**Sagittal**   A vertical plane of section through the body that runs from front to back; also called a **median** plane.

**Sarcomere**   Fundamental unit of muscle contraction; consists of parallel arrays of actin and myosin, contractile protein filaments; chains of linked sarcomeres make up the myofibril.

**Sebum**   The oily secretion found at the base of hair follicles.

**Segmentation**   The act of dividing into segments; a term used to refer to the mixing of food in the small intestine.

**Semen**   Male penile ejaculatory fluid containing sperm and other secretions from the epididymis, prostate gland, seminal vesicles, and bulbourethral gland.

**Semilunar valve**   Valves within the heart that prevent blood in the pulmonary artery and aorta from flowing back into the ventricles.

**Seminiferous tubules**   Coiled tubes in the testes that produce sperm.

**Sensory neuron**   Carries input from sensory receptors to the CNS.

**Sharpey's fibres**   Extensions of collagen fibres that anchor a tendon to its base.

**Sinoatrial node**   The heart's pacemaker; a node within the wall of the right atrium that sends out regular electrical impulses that cause the atria to contract.

**Sinusoids**   Blood channels found within certain organs (liver, spleen, red bone marrow).

**Sphincter**   A ring-shaped muscle that acts as a valve; a circular muscle with concentric rows of fascicles.

**Stratum** (pl. **strata**)   Layer or layers that form any given structure, such as the skin or the retina.

**Substrate**   The substance acted upon and changed by an enzyme.

**Sucrase**   Enzyme that catalyzes the hydrolysis of sucrose into glucose and fructose.

**Sulcus**   A groove (fold) in the surface of the cerebral hemisphere of the brain, separated by gyri.

**Superior**   Above, towards the head; a directional term. See also **cranial**.

**Supination**   A movement of the forearm that turns the palm upward; opposite of **pronation**; movement of the radius around the ulna.

**Suspensory ligament**   Ligament that anchors each ovary laterally to the pelvic wall.

**Suture**   Fixed immovable joint between two bones.

**Synapse**   Junction between two neurons.

**Synergist**   A muscle that complements the action of a prime mover.

**Synovial fluid**   A viscous lubricating (and nutrient) fluid secreted by synovial membrane into bone joints and tendon sheaths.

**Teniae coli** ("ribbons of the colon")   Where the bands of the outer longitudinal muscle layer of the colon are collected; the muscle tone produced by this forms pouches called haustra.

**Testosterone**   Male sex hormone produced by the interstitial (Leydig) cells of the testes (or the adrenals in women); aids sperm production and is necessary for the development of male reproductive organs and secondary sexual characteristics.

**Thoracic cavity**   The cavity formed from the 12 thoracic vertebrae, the 12 pairs of ribs, and the sternum; separated internally into smaller cavities, it houses the chief organs of the circulatory and respiratory systems.

**Thoracic vertebrae**   The 12 bones that make up the middle part of the spine.

**Thyrocalcitonin**   See **calcitonin**.

**Thyroid hormone**   Combination of triiodothyronine and thyroxine released by the thyroid gland; functions as the body's "accelerator pedal" to speed up metabolic rate; helps promote growth and ensures normal functioning of the heart and nervous system.

**Thyroid-stimulating hormone (TSH)**   Hormone released by the anterior pituitary gland. It stimulates the release of thyroid hormone by the thyroid gland.

**Thyroxine**   Hormone released by the thyroid gland. It increases metabolism and the sensitivity of the cardiovascular system to the nervous system.

**Trabeculae**   Tiny spikes of bone tissue surrounded by calcified bone matrix; predominantly found in the interior of spongy bone.

**Tricuspid valve**   The right atrioventricular heart valve.

**Triiodothyronine**   Hormone released by the thyroid gland; increases metabolism and the sensitivity of the cardiovascular system.

**Trypsin**   Enzyme found in pancreatic juice that breaks down proteins.

**Tunica adventitia**   The tough fibrous outer layer of an arterial wall; consists mainly of collagen fibres and elastic tissue.

**Tunica intima**   The inner lining of the lumen of an artery.

**Tunica media**   The middle, and thickest, layer of an arterial wall; consists of smooth muscle and elastic tissue.

**Umbilical cord**   A tube that connects the embryo and the placenta; carries oxygen and nutrients to the embryo, and carbon dioxide and nitrogenous waste matter from the embryo.

**Unipennate**   A pennate muscle where fascicles are attached to one side of the tendon (e.g., extensor digitorum longus).

**Urea**   Nitrogenous waste product produced by the chemical breakdown of proteins in the body; excreted in urine.

**Urethra**   The duct through which urine (and semen in the male) passes from the bladder to the exterior.

**Urine**   Excretory waste fluid produced by the kidneys; consists mainly of water, urea, salts, phosphates, sulphates, creatinine, and uric acid.

**Uterus**   A hollow, muscular organ situated behind the bladder that houses, nourishes, and protects the developing fetus.

**Utricle**   The larger of the two balance-detectors in the ear.

**Vas deferens**   The excretory duct of each testicle, extending between the epididymis of each testicle and the ejaculatory duct.

**Vein**   A blood vessel that carries blood towards the heart; the blood is usually deoxygenated, although the pulmonary veins carry newly oxygenated blood to the left ventricle of the heart.

**Ventral**   Directional term; towards the front of the body. See also **anterior**.

**Ventricular systole**   Contraction of the ventricles during the cardiac cycle, causing the ventricle to empty of blood.

**Vesico-uterine pouch**   Fold of peritoneum that forms behind the bladder and in front of the neck of the uterus.

**Vestibule**   A cavity, chamber, or channel serving as an approach or entrance to another cavity; refers to the central chamber of the labyrinth of the middle ear.

**Villi**   Tiny fingerlike processes in the mucosa of the small intestine that increase the available surface area.

**Virus**   Any of numerous kinds of intracellular parasite characterized by a bare core of nucleic acid (RNA or DNA) enclosed in a protein shell (the capsid). Viruses utilize host cells' constituents for their own replication and may cause disease and infectious spread in this way.

**Viscera**   The internal organs of the body.

**Visceral peritoneum**   The serous membrane that covers the abdominal organs.

**Visual association area**   Area of the brain (surrounding the primary visual cortex) that compares incoming visual information with previously seen images, allowing recognition of familiar objects/faces.

**White pulp**   Area of the spleen involved in the immune response; consists of suspended lymphocytes that generate antibody-producing cells.